Preventing drowning: an implementation guide

World Health Organization

Preventing drowning: an implementation guide

ISBN 978-92-4-151193-3

Suggested citation.
Preventing drowning: an implementation guide. Geneva: World Health Organization; 2017. Licence: CC BY-NC-SA 3.0 IGO.

Cataloguing-in-Publication (CIP) data.
CIP data are available at http://apps.who.int/iris.

Printed in Spain.

Made possible through funding from Bloomberg Philanthropies.

Contents

Foreword

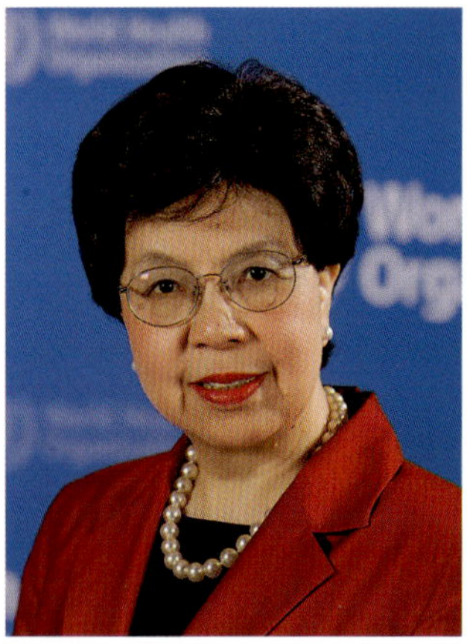

Margaret Chan,
Director-General,
World Health Organization

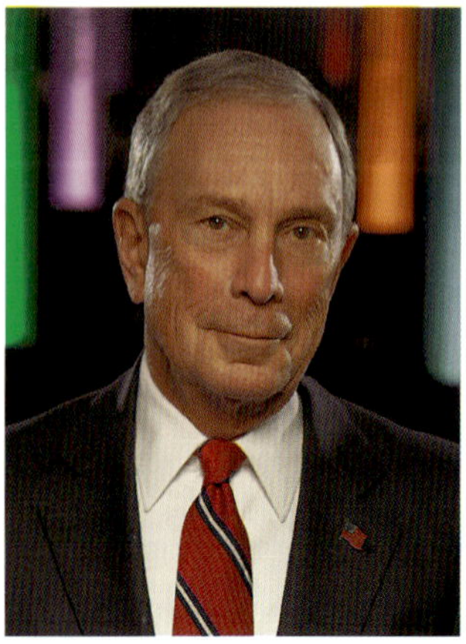

Michael R Bloomberg,
WHO Global Ambassador for Noncommunicable Diseases

Far too many people around the world know the pain of losing a loved one to drowning. Each year almost 360 000 people die from drowning – over 90% of them in low- and middle-income countries. More than half of these deaths are among those younger than 25, with children aged under 5 facing the greatest risk. Drowning is the third leading cause of death worldwide for those aged from 5 to 14. Despite these tragic facts, drowning prevention gets relatively little attention and few resources.

There is far more we can do to prevent drowning. Global commitments made as part of the Sustainable Development Goals, for example, cannot be met as long as this preventable cause of death is left largely unchecked. All of us – policy-makers, parents, non-profit organizations, businesses and concerned citizens – can help prevent drowning. Explaining how is the goal of this guide.

Building on the World Health Organization's 2014 *Global report on drowning*, the following pages provide practical, step-by-step guidance on how to implement 10 effective measures to prevent drowning. They range from community-based solutions, such as day care for children and barriers controlling access to water, to effective national policies and legislation around water safety, including setting and enforcing boating, shipping and ferry regulations. Data show that all of these solutions can help save lives.

The more we work together to implement the measures outlined in this guide, the more lives can be saved. We urge all concerned to adopt as many of the interventions and strategies as their resources will allow, and to protect those most vulnerable without delay.

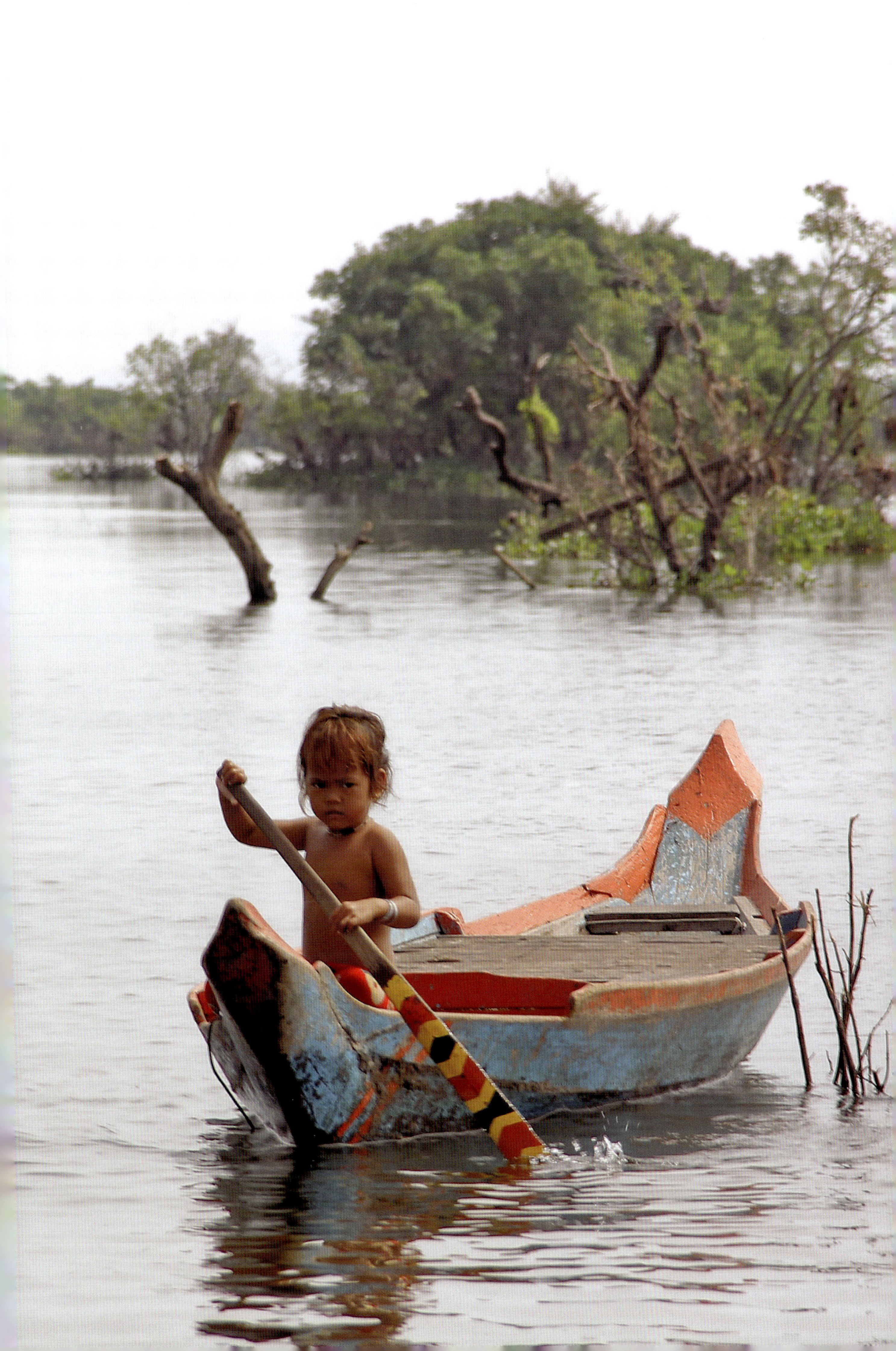

Acknowledgements

The World Health Organization would like to thank the following contributors and reviewers who provided the content and expert feedback essential to the production of this guide. The World Health Organization is very grateful for their generosity in terms of both time and effort.

Executive Editor: David Meddings

Contributors: Elena Altieri, Joost Bierens, Erin Cassell, Andrew Gissing, Jonathan Guevarra, Adnan Hyder, David Jardine-Smith, Olive Kobusingye, Michael Linnan, David Meddings, Joan Ozanne-Smith, Aminur Rahman, Len Roueche, Justin Scarr, Elizabeth Towner, Shirin Wadhwaniya and Roberta Weisbrod.

Reviewers: Olakunle Alonge, Peter Barss, Stephen Beerman, Elizabeth Bennett, Lauren S Blum, Ruth Brenner, Tessa Clemens, Ross Cox, Shelley Dalke, Jac Dendle, Richard C Franklin, Daniel Graham, Robert Greif, Gopalkrishna Gururaj, John Leech, Ashok Mahapatra, Kulanthayan KC Mani, Thomas Mecrow, Julie Mytton, Puspa Raj Pant, Jonathon Passmore, John Pearn, Cuong Pham Viet, Linda Quan, Fazlur Rahman, Daniel Ryan, David Szpilman, Chadia Wannous, John Waterhouse, Steve Wills and Stephen Yeo.

The report benefited from the input of a number of other people. Angela Burton edited the report. Rebecca Bavinger and Kelly Larson from Bloomberg Philanthropies contributed thoughtful reviews. Ingvar Berg, Justin Sempsrott and Theo Verhoeven provided additional guidance. Other WHO staff that reviewed the report were Alison Harvey, Etienne Krug, Margie Peden, Laura Sminkey and Tami Toroyan.

Finally the World Health Organization wishes to thank Bloomberg Philanthropies for its generous financial support for the development and publication of this report.

Abbreviations

AWSC	Australian Water Safety Council
BHIS	Bangladesh Health and Injury Survey
CPR	cardiopulmonary resuscitation
ERC	European Resuscitation Council
IAMSAR	International Aeronautical and Maritime Search and Rescue
IMO	International Maritime Organization
IMRF	International Maritime Rescue Federation
KAP	knowledge, attitudes and practice (survey)
MSV	Marine Safety Victoria
NGO	nongovernmental organization
NOAA	National Aeronautical and Atmospheric Administration
PFD	personal flotation device
SAR	search and rescue
SDGs	Sustainable Development Goals
SoLiD	Saving Lives from Drowning
UNICEF	United Nations Children's Fund
WHO	World Health Organization

Introduction

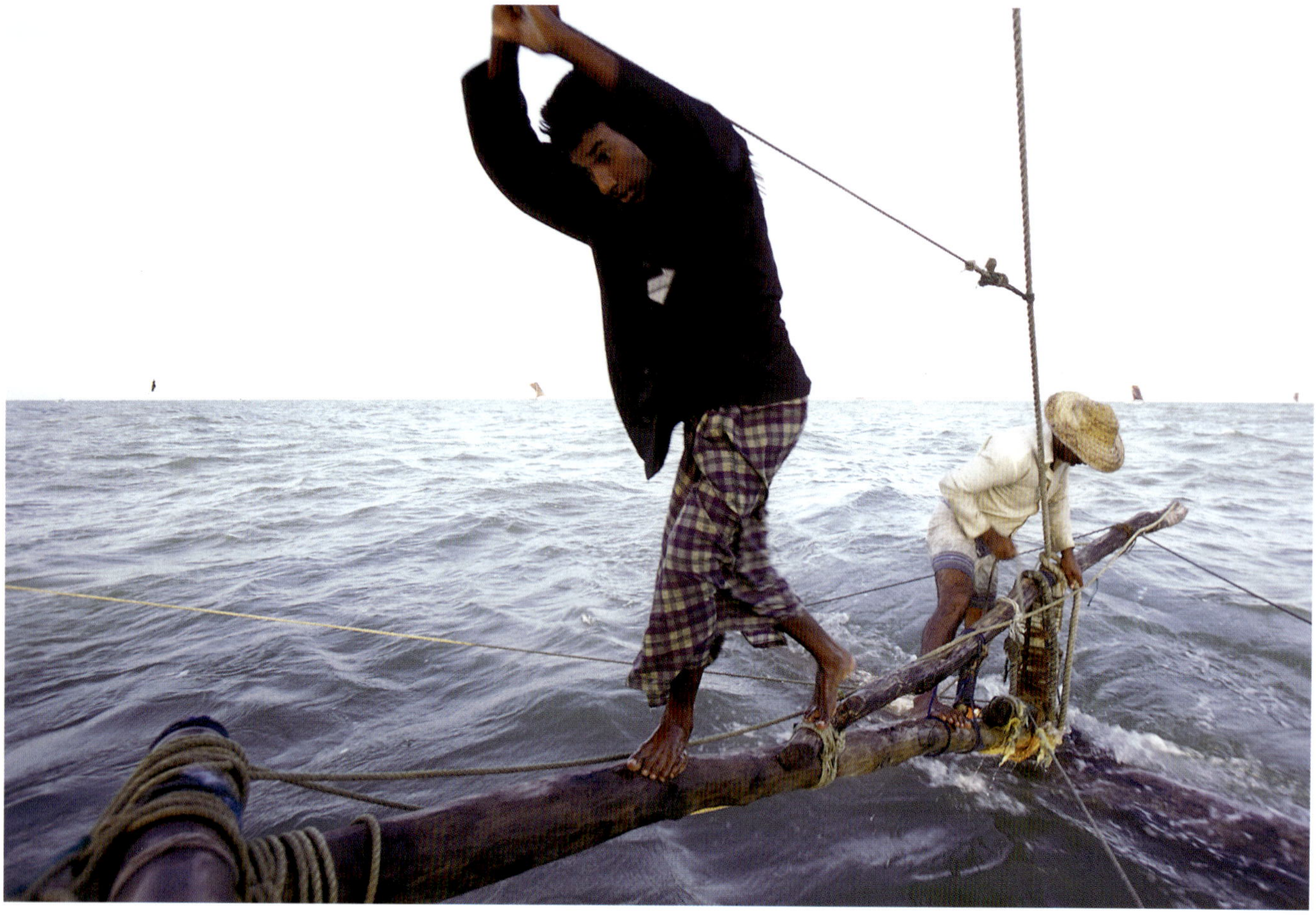

This guide provides practical steps to reduce drowning – one of the world's most preventable, neglected and pressing public health issues. Through 10 evidence-based interventions and strategies it is designed to help drowning-prevention practitioners – from nongovernmental organizations (NGOs) and researchers to government officials and policy-makers – approach drowning prevention in a strategic, evidence-based and multisectoral way. It also highlights ways to harness public awareness and engagement to strengthen drowning prevention interventions.

At national or community level, drowning can be prevented through implementing six selected **interventions** and four "cross-cutting" **implementation strategies** that underpin them.[1] These are:

Interventions

Install barriers controlling access to water

Provide safe places (for example a day-care centre) away from water for pre-school children, with capable child care

Teach school-age children swimming and water safety skills

Train bystanders in safe rescue and resuscitation

Set and enforce safe boating, shipping and ferry regulations

Build resilience and manage flood risks and other hazards locally and nationally

Strategies

Strengthen public awareness of drowning through strategic communications

Promote multisectoral collaboration

Develop a national water safety plan

Advance drowning prevention through data collection and well-designed studies

These **interventions** and **strategies** were selected as the best evidence-based ways to prevent drowning in the *Global report on drowning: preventing a leading killer (1)* – though many of them are more commonly used in high-income countries than the low- and middle-income countries where 90% of the global drowning burden lies.

1 This guide includes the same 10 actions to prevent drowning contained in the *Global report on drowning*, but for simplicity this guide groups them as "strategies" and "interventions" rather than "community-based actions", "policies and legislation" and "research".

How to use this guide

In resource-poor settings where educational levels may be low, it is important to understand how people perceive drowning before introducing interventions.

As a first step, a **situational assessment** will help decide which strategies and interventions are likely to make the most impact on drowning in your community, region or country, based on your available resources (the more interventions you can implement, the more successful they are collectively likely to be).

Once you have selected your **interventions**, consider the potential benefit of each of our four recommended **strategies** upon your chosen interventions and implement as many as possible. These strategies can strengthen both an intervention's impact and the evidence base of the drowning prevention field.

Examples of how strategies can enhance the effectiveness of interventions include the following scenarios:

- A village-based programme to establish **child care for pre-school children** in a setting with no prior experience of it is far more likely to be effective if it **raises public awareness** among villagers about risks to pre-school children who have no constant adult supervision.
- A programme to **teach school-age children swimming and water safety skills** can benefit from **collaboration** with the education sector, which can provide venues for safe training and teachers trained to provide swim skills training.
- A national effort to strengthen enforcement of **safe boating, shipping and ferry regulations** is far more likely to be successful if it engages a **multisectoral** range of stakeholders, is accompanied by communication efforts to **raise public awareness**, and is part of a regulatory framework referred to in **national water safety plans**.

In resource-poor settings where educational levels may be low, it is important to understand how people perceive drowning before introducing interventions, including what local people see as the cause of drowning and appropriate ways to treat and prevent it. In drowning prevention partnerships and/or interventions in at-risk communities, donors and technical partners must ensure that their needs and interests do not overshadow those of the countries, communities or organizations being supported. If not managed carefully, the negative impacts of ignoring this principle can include poor results and increased drowning risk.

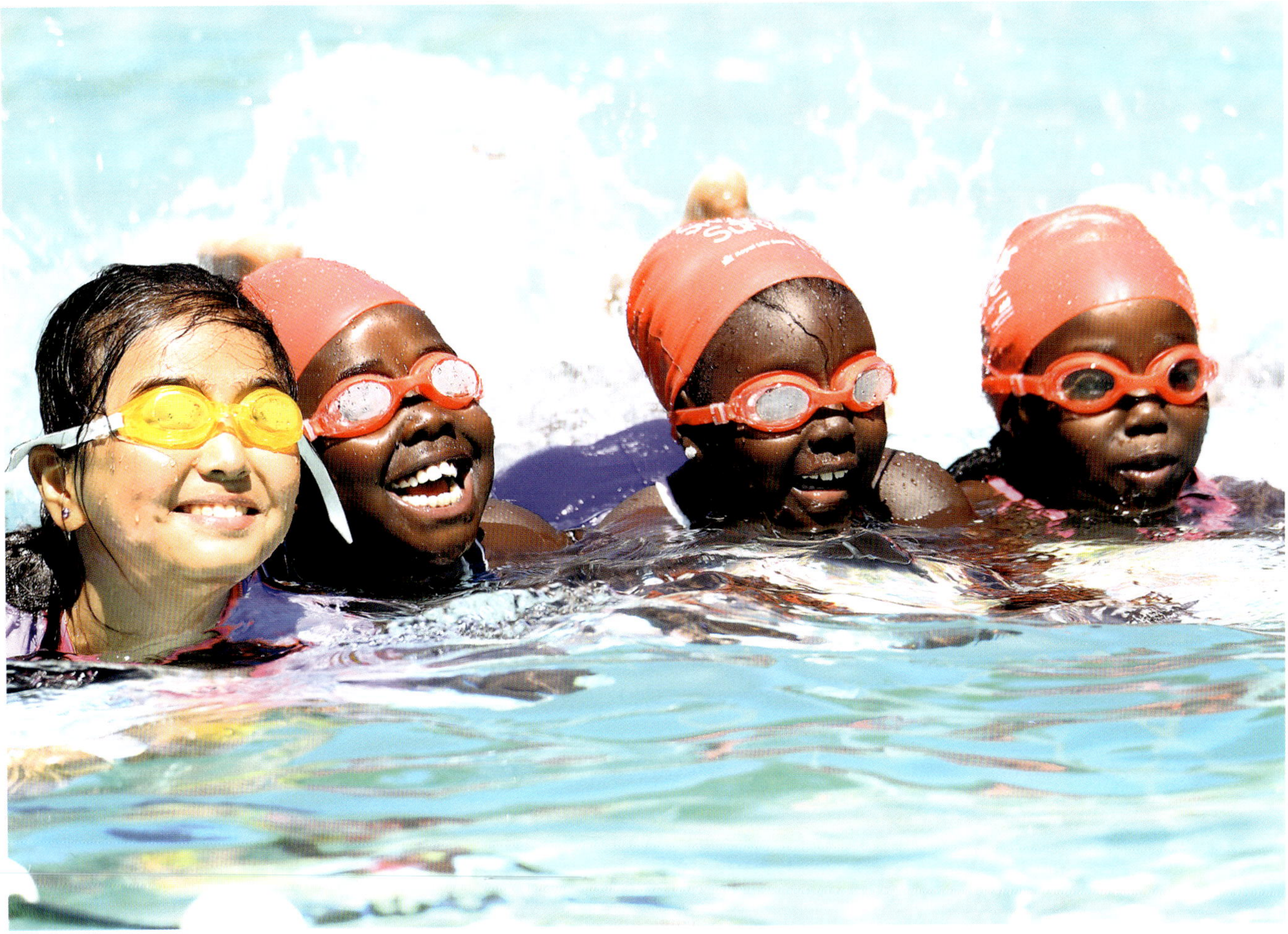

As the guidance contained in this resource needs to be relevant for those working in a mix of international, national or community-level contexts, it sometimes highlights considerations more relevant to one of these contexts than the others.

What this guide contains

Section 1 sets out guidance on carrying out a situational assessment – a prerequisite for preventing drowning in any setting, and one that reveals the local drowning profile and current efforts to deal with drowning prevention. It includes a stakeholder and resource analysis.

Section 2 provides guidance on the six different interventions to prevent drowning.

Section 3 provides guidance on the four cross-cutting implementation strategies that support the six interventions, including a snapshot of the need addressed, the benefits of the intervention or strategy, and the key steps to implementing it.

Section 1

Situational assessments

Implementing any intervention to prevent drowning begins with a situational assessment to establish a number of key facts that are essential to proper prioritization and planning. Situational assessments maximize effective implementation of all 10 drowning prevention interventions and strategies in this guide. Some of the strategies (for example, developing a national water safety plan) overlap with the steps described here.

What should a situational assessment do?

A situational assessment should answer the following questions:

- What are the most pressing drowning issues and their context?
- What is the at-risk population's understanding of the causes of drowning and how to prevent it?
- Which intervention could be delivered to address these issues?
- Is the intervention targeted at the most appropriate location and group?
- Are there other relevant efforts underway?
- Is there a regulatory or legislative framework that applies – and if so, is it effectively enforced?
- Which stakeholder groups will have an impact on how effectively the intervention is implemented (note that some stakeholders may oppose the intervention)?
- Where are the resources – human and financial – to implement the intervention, and can these be increased if the intervention needs to be scaled up?
- Does the intervention address drowning disparities among different population groups and promote equity?

Situational assessments maximize effective implementation of all 10 drowning prevention interventions and strategies in this guide.

Five components of a situational assessment

1 Review available data

2 Assess current efforts

3 Assess existing policy and regulation

4 Identify relevant stakeholders

5 Assess required human and financial resources

Each of these components is essential but a balance must be made between collecting enough information and not expending too many resources upon it. For example, the costs of collecting new data must be weighed against using existing (limited) data to guide action that may save lives.

Review available data

Reviewing available data helps decide what populations should be targeted and what type of intervention is likely to have the greatest impact, be it at local, regional or national level.

See page 67

A range of sources may have data on drowning. Formal requests for access to some data sources may be necessary, which emphasizes the importance of establishing collaborative relationships with stakeholders, including government (see Promote multisectoral collaboration). The following sources of drowning data should be considered:

- Some **national as well as state or provincial health data collection systems** will have injury surveillance systems that can provide data on fatal and non-fatal drownings.
- **Vital registration systems** can provide vital statistics reports with cause of death information, although these systems may have important deficiencies in low- and middle-income settings, particularly for locations where drowning rates may be higher.[2]
- **Surveys** on drowning may have been carried out by researchers, lifesaving associations, NGOs or government agencies.
- Some countries have **dedicated drowning information databases.**
- A range of local or national authorities may maintain records or have information on drowning or water hazards, including hospitals, the police, coast guard, water transport agencies and disaster risk reduction authorities.
- Other, less formal sources can help guide understanding of drowning, including media reports (**traditional, digital** and **social media** tend to report information on the circumstances of drowning which may not otherwise be available), and **local people**.

Data gathered from these sources should be collated and presented in a clear, easily understood format. If data are insufficient it may be necessary to carry out a dedicated survey to establish a drowning profile. WHO has produced guidance for developing and conducting surveys at community level *(2)* (though numbers of drownings in small areas are likely to be low).

The review of available data should provide answers to the following questions regardless of whether your intervention is implemented at local, regional or national level:

- What is the age, sex, race, ethnicity, occupation and income level of those most likely to drown?

2 Vital registration systems register births and deaths, issue birth and death certificates and compile and disseminate vital statistics. The percentage of all deaths occurring that are captured by these systems is variable. WHO regards 85% coverage of deaths and higher as desirable and does not report on data provided by such systems if coverage is below 70% of deaths. Countries where vital registration systems cover a lower percentage of deaths tend to be low- and middle-income countries, and within these, deaths within rural areas – where drowning rates tend to be higher – are less likely to be recorded than deaths in urban areas.

- Where and when do drownings occur?
- What are the water bodies in which people most frequently drown?
- Are data available about the activities taking place at the time of drowning (e.g. while working, or at leisure or play)? If so, what do they reveal?
- Is the at-risk population changing over time?
- Is the risk itself changing over time?

Assess current efforts

Assessing current drowning prevention programmes and practice reveals work already underway, where it is taking place, by whom, and the resources applied to it. The assessment can also yield important information about the effectiveness of these interventions, and any gaps in knowledge and practice.

Assessing current efforts requires two approaches:

- A **desk review** of research reports, published papers and programme evaluations. Some of these may have already come to light during the review of available data. Peer-reviewed papers and programme evaluations in particular can provide comprehensive information.
- **Key informants** should be identified and interviewed. Key informants may include international organizations, relevant ministries, academic or research institutions, NGOs, health-care practitioners, local authorities and community leaders, and local media.

If data are insufficient it may be necessary to carry out a dedicated survey to establish a drowning profile.

Assess existing policy and regulation

This relatively straightforward part of the assessment is primarily done through a desk review, alongside interviews with key informants, possibly from several sectors. At a minimum, the assessment should clarify the following:

- The existence of any laws, regulatory frameworks or policies relevant to the intervention being considered (it may be helpful to tap into international standards to help inform appropriate interventions and ensure their effectiveness, for example on the floating properties of lifejackets).
- Which entities have legal jurisdiction and responsibility for enforcement of relevant laws and regulatory frameworks related to drowning prevention.

Depending on the scope of the intervention(s) being considered, it may also be appropriate for this part of the assessment to develop an understanding of the following:

- Important gaps in existing policy and regulation relevant to the intervention(s) (it may be necessary to look at policies and regulations in use elsewhere to identify these gaps).
- The degree to which measures that are a part of regulatory frameworks or legal requirements are actively enforced.

Stakeholder analysis begins by compiling a list of stakeholders relevant to the successful implementation of the drowning prevention intervention.

As with the assessment of current efforts, an opportunity exists to use this component of the situational assessment to develop multisectoral collaboration – for example, ensuring a new law mandating the use of a lifejacket[3] can be supported by the media in promoting awareness; lifesaving organizations in showing people how to use them; government public awareness adverts; and the police by enforcing the new law. This can be particularly helpful if there are gaps in existing policy and regulation, or failings in enforcement.

Determine relevant stakeholders

Stakeholder analysis begins by compiling a list of stakeholders relevant to the successful implementation of the drowning prevention intervention. The method for doing this depends on the setting and the intervention(s) being considered. You may use a "snowballing" technique whereby you identify one set of stakeholders and then ask them who they think other stakeholders might be.

An approach that broadly categorizes stakeholders may be helpful, as illustrated in Table 1. For example, if an intervention to provide day care for pre-school children is being considered, and the intention is to implement this with a very strong research component, then a university or research institution will very likely be a stakeholder. It is important to note that stakeholders can be an important source of learning and can greatly extend the skillsets involved in a drowning prevention effort. For example, stakeholders can share their expertise in marketing, manufacturing, technology development and preparing business strategies, which may help scale-up the project.

3 This guide uses the term "lifejacket" instead of "personal flotation device" or "PFD" as used in the *Global report on drowning.*

Table 1: Example stakeholders that may be identified by stakeholder analysis[a]

Intervention	Stakeholder type		
	Authorities (government departments and agents, certifying bodies)	Nongovernmental associations, research or academic institutions, industry/business, water recreation facilities, watersports societies	Target population
Install barriers controlling access to water	Community leaders; municipal governments; national and regional governments; public health workers involved in home visiting	Lifesaving organizations; child health NGOs; rural development NGOs; media	Parents; homeowners with pools; families; community members (particularly those most vulnerable)
Provide safe places (for example, a day-care centre) away from water for pre-school children, with capable child care	Community leaders; municipal governments; national and regional governments; school and pre-school authorities	Women's groups; lifesaving societies; child development and education NGOs; rural development NGOs	Parents; families (particularly those most vulnerable)
Teach school-age children swimming and water safety skills	Community leaders; religious and traditional leaders; municipal governments; national and regional governments; teachers; school nurses	Lifesaving organizations and/or the Red Cross movement; swimming clubs or associations; child health NGOs; rural development NGOs; research institutes	Parents; school children; religious and traditional leaders; health professionals
Train bystanders in safe rescue and resuscitation	Community leaders; municipal governments; national and regional governments; teachers, health-care providers	Lifesaving organizations and/or Red Cross movement; swimming clubs or associations; associations for high-risk occupations; media; resuscitation and first aid agencies; ambulance services; police and firefighters	Parents; school children; health professionals; vessel operators; search and rescue personnel
Set and enforce safe boating, shipping and ferry regulations	Community leaders; national governments; coast guard; maritime police; police	Vessel operator associations; lifesaving organizations and/or Red Cross movement; associations for high-risk occupations and recreation; media; vessel builders	Vessel operators; search and rescue personnel; recreational boaters
Build resilience and manage flood risks and other hazards locally and nationally	Community leaders; national, regional and local levels of government; national weather monitoring entities; flood mapping services; national disaster risk reduction councils	Lifesaving organizations and/or Red Cross movement; associations for high-risk occupations and recreation; media Researchers, geographers, engineers, meteorologists etc.	Search and rescue personnel; communities with high vulnerability to disaster; general population

[a] This table does not represent an exhaustive list of all possible stakeholders.

Once a list of potential stakeholders has been compiled, strategic attention should be given to the following questions:

- **How critical is this stakeholder** to the successful implementation of the intervention?
- **Are they predisposed to engaging?** If not, what needs to be invested to secure their engagement or reduce any resistance?
- **What role can they play to enhance the intervention?**
- **What are the benefits to the drowning prevention effort and the stakeholder?**

The stakeholder analysis may also indicate whether an intervention is likely to fail – if critical stakeholders are not likely to engage it may be advisable to re-think the intervention.

Determine human and financial resources

This part of the situational assessment determines the level of financial and human resources available for the intervention, and can reveal opportunities for wider collaboration. An argument that may be useful in widening the range of potential collaborators is that investment in drowning prevention has the potential to save money elsewhere in the system, since national estimates of annual costs of drowning (where studied) have been estimated to run from US$ 85 million to US$ 4.1 billion *(1)*.

The evidence base for drowning prevention activities is emerging slowly... but everyone concerned with drowning prevention can help it expand through rigorously monitoring and evaluating their own interventions.

The analysis also has importance for longer term sustainability and scaling up of the intervention. When considering financial resources it is desirable to diversify funding wherever possible, in particular getting funding from national governments instead of international donors and asking for small amounts from stakeholders to help with "buy in".

Building human resource capacity involves, among other things, developing, implementing and learning from well-designed research and cultivating local understanding and knowledge through small interventions before bringing such interventions to scale.

Monitoring and evaluation

The evidence base for drowning prevention activities is emerging slowly – especially in low- and middle-income countries – but everyone concerned with drowning prevention can help it expand through rigorously monitoring and evaluating their own interventions. This means collecting and analysing information about interventions; identifying problems and providing feedback; processing and analysing data promptly; and passing the results to those in a position to take action.

Monitoring requires demonstrating the outcomes of the 10 interventions and strategies in this guide via specific sets of indicators (where possible, potential indicators are suggested for some interventions and strategies). In general, these should reveal if the interventions and strategies reached the intended populations; were delivered as intended (and, if not, whether adjustments made to the interventions and strategies were appropriate to the local context, or had a negative impact on the outcome); and if they were perceived as acceptable by the communities to which they were offered.

For example, indicators for a day-care centre could include: the number of days for which care was available; the hours this care was available for each day; the age of children attending; and the number and training level of supervisors. Monitoring a day-care centre as part of an intervention to prevent drowning means evaluators might want to know, for example, the proportion of the population for whom the day-care centre is available; the proportion of the eligible population attending the centre; and the number of drowning or near-drowning cases before and since introduction of the day-care centre.

As with improving monitoring and evaluation systems, shared indicators should be disaggregated by sex and age groups, disability and other demographic characteristics where relevant.

See page 89

Specific monitoring and evaluation considerations are given for each intervention and strategy where available, and further information on monitoring and evaluation is provided in our research strategy section (see Research).

Section 2

Six interventions to prevent drowning

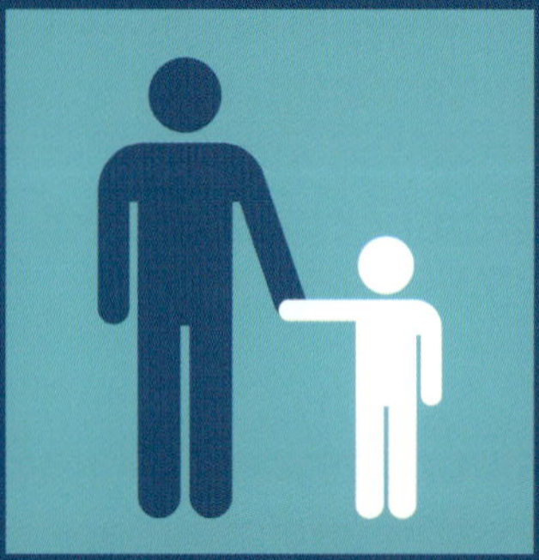

1

Provide safe places away from water for pre-school children

Page 15

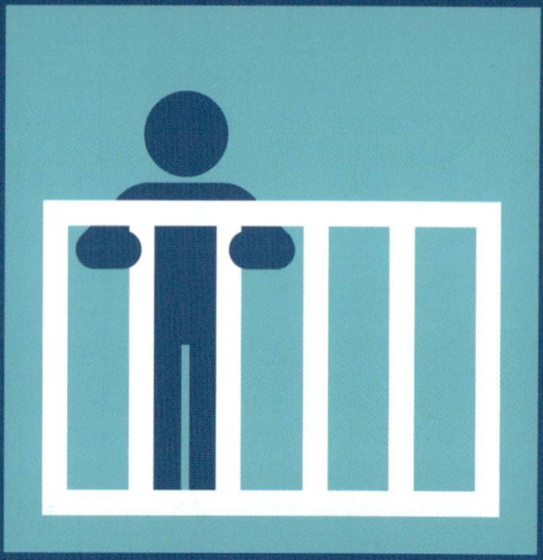

2

Install barriers controlling access to water

Page 22

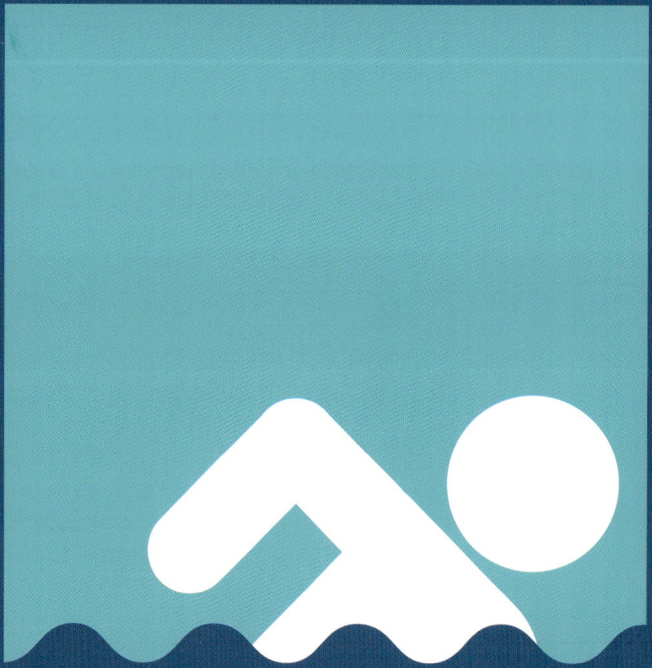

3

Teach school-age children (aged over 6 years) swimming and water safety skills

Page 30

4

Build resilience and manage flood risks and other hazards
Page 41

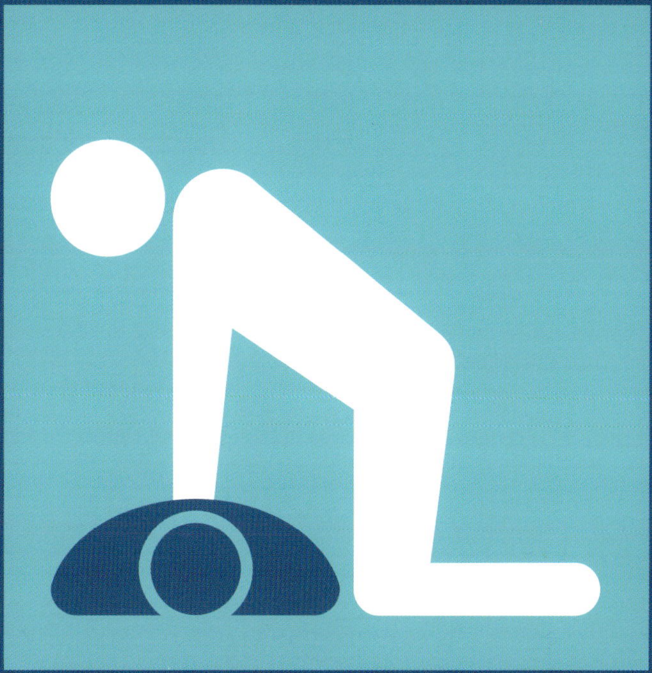

5

Train bystanders in safe rescue and resuscitation
Page 47

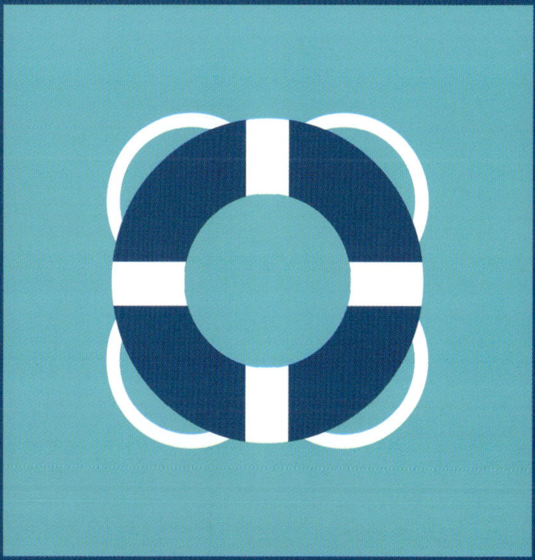

6

Set and enforce safe boating, shipping and ferry regulations
Page 54

1

Provide safe places away from water for pre-school children, with capable childcare

Globally *(1)* children aged 1–4 years are the most vulnerable to drowning as they are mobile and may fall into open or unobstructed water bodies from which they cannot get out *(3)*. Lack of parental awareness about the risks and prevention of childhood drowning, inadequate supervision and extensive exposure to water bodies are notable risk factors for drowning in this age group.

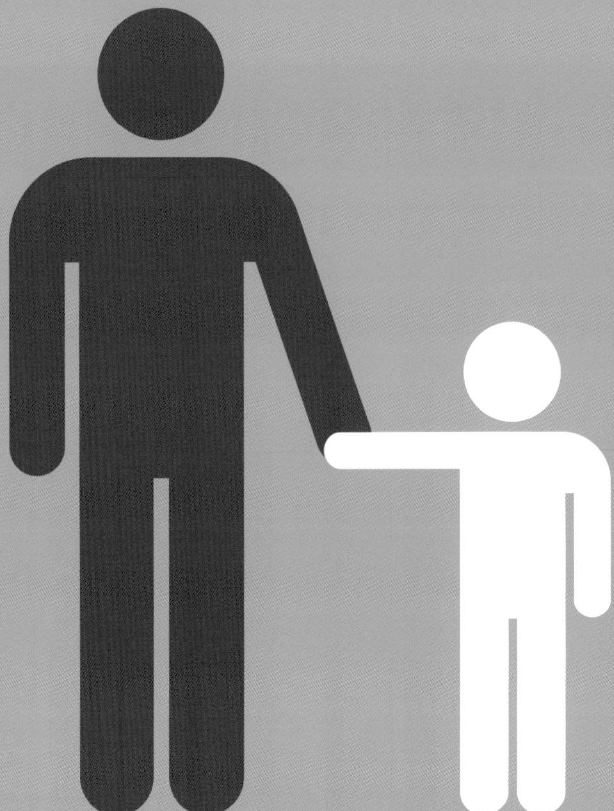

Benefits of safe places away from water for pre-school children, with capable child care

In low- and middle-income countries (and also in many high-income countries) childhood drowning tends to occur during guardians' busy hours, when they are doing housework or other daily tasks. Community-based institutional supervision of children during the hours when they are most likely to drown is a useful intervention to protect them from drowning and may also ensure that older children are not burdened by supervision of siblings and are free to attend school. However, in most low- and middle-income countries (unlike high-income countries) such care is almost non-existent.

One exception is Bangladesh, where, in order to prevent childhood drowning, a community day-care centre programme locally known as *"Anchal"* was trialled and found to be culturally and socially acceptable, and both effective and cost-effective.[4] The study showed that children participating in the programme had lower fatal drowning rates than those who did not participate *(4)*. Village-based, supervised child-care programmes for drowning prevention also exist in south India and Cambodia *(1)*.

Community-based institutional supervision of children during the hours when they are most likely to drown is a useful intervention to protect them from drowning.

While such centres are cost-effective in terms of drowning prevention and other early childhood development gains, long-term funding can be hard to secure (in the case of the Anchal programme, when donor funding ended and the programme closed, there was a negative effect on the community). Investigators are currently exploring how such centres can therefore be established sustainably in low- and middle-income settings. The Bangladesh Anchal and SwimSafe (BASS) project is examining, among other issues, how day-care arrangements can be established in a financially and socially sustainable manner in a low-income context.

4 In low- and middle-income countries prevalence of infectious diseases that spread rapidly among children gathered together is high. Parents are taught to keep sick children at home and day-care attendants receive training to minimize exposures to children and themselves. A similar approach is implemented in Anchals in Bangladesh, and should be adopted by any activity that brings young children together in groups on a regular basis.

Implementing safe places away from water for pre-school children

⇩ Step one

Assess the current day-care provision situation

See page 5

Include in your situational assessment any government programmes relating to early childhood development or pre-formal schooling. Early childhood development programmes differ by country – for example, the Philippines government runs a scheme to provide day care for children aged 3 years or older until they go to school.

⇩ Step two

Define target group

Defining which children will benefit most from child care should be determined based on drowning patterns in the community and relevant social and cultural factors identified by the situational assessment. In most countries, children in child care are pre-school age. However "school age" may differ from one community to another. Further, in some communities, sending infants (those under the age of 12 months) to a day-care centre may be socially acceptable, while in other communities it may not. In such cases, 1–4 years may be more appropriate.

⇩ Step three

Establish and equip the day-care centre

In many countries the physical and staffing requirements for day-care centres will already be regulated and should be consulted. Day-care centres need to be a convenient walking distance from home, with an acceptable ratio of children per trained carer,[5] with one or two support staff.

The day-care centre should be large enough to comfortably accommodate the children and allow activities, including games. It should have good lighting and ventilation, and be suitable for children in all types of weather. Entrances and exits should be controlled using door-barriers (made from locally available materials such as bamboo or timber) so that children, especially younger ones, cannot leave the room unaccompanied. It should be a clean environment with safe water and sanitation, facilities for breastfeeding mothers, and the floor should be clean. If a community building is not

5 Carer-to-child ratios can vary widely depending on context, for example: a country's income level; the care setting (government-run centre, family-provided day care, emergency situation etc.); children's ages. Intervention trials such as Bangladesh's *Anchal* and SwimSafe programmes are currently exploring optimal staffing ratios that maximize drowning risk reduction with overall programme sustainability.

available, a room large enough to comfortably accommodate the group in the house of a carer (and which meets the above criteria) could be used, reducing programme costs.

Day care may prevent drowning and also provides the opportunity to improve early childhood development. Children should be engaged in fun and interesting activities appropriate for their age while at the centre, which should be sufficiently equipped with early learning materials and safe toys to stimulate physical, intellectual, linguistic, social and emotional development.

⇩ Step four

Select and train carers

Day care may prevent drowning and also provides the opportunity to improve early childhood development.

Potential carers should have as high a level of education as possible and preferably come from the community that will use the day care provided. In low- and middle-income countries where background checks are weak or non-existent, community involvement in carer selection may be useful in the interests of child protection ("good character" references and ongoing monitoring from community leaders may be the only alternative to the background screening system used in high-income countries). A local committee may select the carers using criteria such as educational status, keenness for the role, and where necessary the ability to provide a room in their home as the venue for the day-care centre. After selection, carers should be given hands-on training in child supervision, early childhood development stimulations and early learning – particularly for children aged 3 years and over. Carers should be given regular refresher training in order to retain these skills.

Caregivers need to be motivated and empowered – doing so will increase their likelihood of working with enthusiasm. This may require incentives such as further training or provision of a specific role within the community. In rural areas where women get little opportunity to earn an income, selecting them as carers may offer them a worthwhile income opportunity. Any financial remuneration should take into account the local cost of living, as well as how programme costs will be sustained through involvement of partners (e.g. government, community, external funders, or partnerships involving a mix of these).

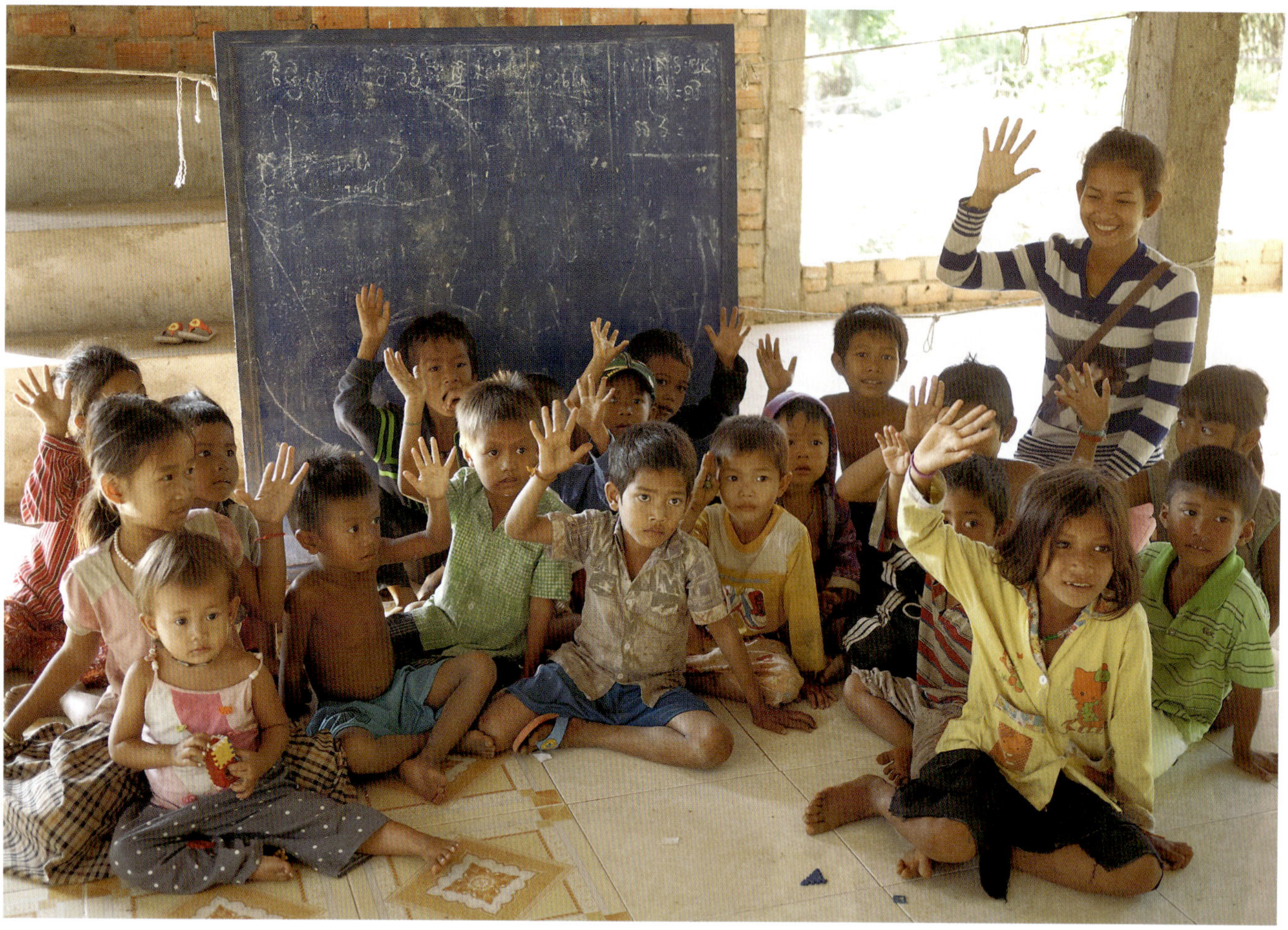

Engaging the community is crucial for successful day-care centre implementation.

Step five

Engage the community and share information with parents

Engaging the community is crucial for successful day-care centre implementation and must be addressed in the situational assessment as part of the stakeholder analysis. The community should be informed about the importance of a day-care centre for drowning and injury prevention. Local committees can be very useful, involving community leaders and elders such as local authority officials, school teachers, religious leaders and other informal leaders influential in the community. The committee may be engaged in activities such as venue and carer selection, and provide oversight of day-care activities.

Parents should attend regular meetings, moderated by the carer/s. During the meeting, parents may be reminded about the importance of keeping children in a day-care centre and learn about their children's development. During these meetings, parents can also be educated on issues such as the safety of their children, including drowning prevention, child nutrition and health and hygiene, including hand washing and latrine use.

⇩ Step six

Ensure supervision and monitoring of carers

To ensure activities are carried out professionally and sustainably, regular supervision and monitoring of day care by a trained supervisor is essential. Supervisors should be trained alongside carers on the activities of the day-care centre and should receive further training on supervising and monitoring both the carers and the physical environment of the centre (including equipment, protocols, training, evaluation and impact of the centre). One supervisor may cover many day-care centres. The supervisor should use a structured checklist to monitor these aspects. The aims of supervision are to improve carer performance, identify carers who are markedly above or below the normal level of quality, and ensure the centre is well maintained and fully functional.

⇩ Step seven

Consider ways to scale-up and improve sustainability of day-care provision

See page 67

Scalability and sustainability of this type of programme is a great concern in low- and middle-income countries – in most cases day-care programmes end when external funding runs out. Integration with other established national activities – including education curricula or child welfare activities – will improve scalability and sustainability of day-care activities and is therefore paramount (see Promote multisectoral collaboration for more on integrating drowning prevention into multiple sectors' activities). Investigating the possibility of day-care users contributing to operational costs should be explored.

⇩ Step eight

Monitor and evaluate

Monitoring a day-care centre as part of an intervention to prevent drowning may mean evaluating, for example, the proportion of the population for whom the day-care centre is available; the proportion of the eligible population attending the centre; and the number of drowning or near-drowning cases before and since introduction of the day-care centre.

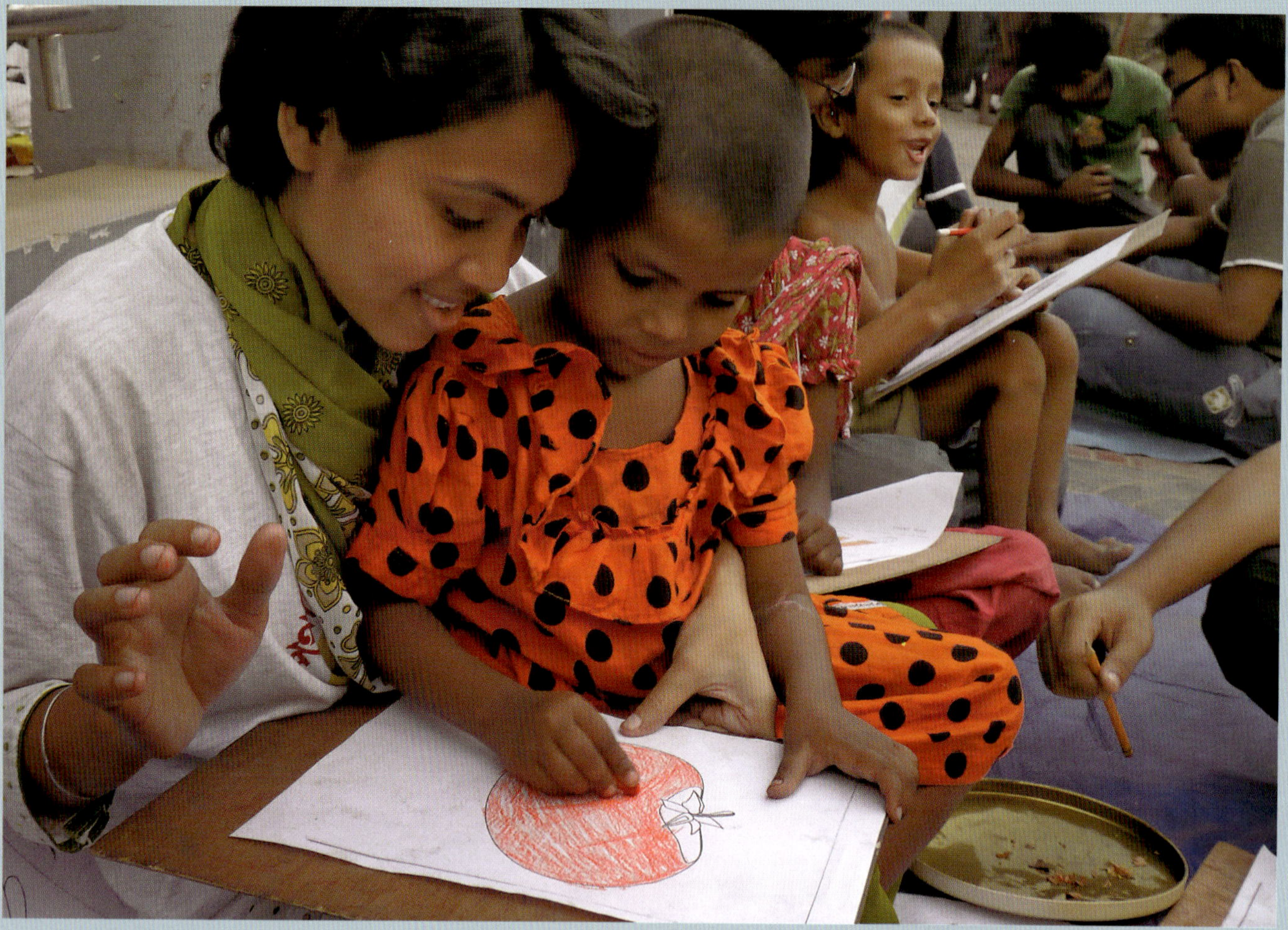

Case study

Bereaved parents champion day care as a way to prevent children from drowning, Bangladesh

Sayed Ali and Shilpee Khatun (not featured in the image above) live in Sherpur district, Bangladesh. They lost their son, Selim, in 2011 when he was just 4 years old. Selim was playing beside a pond near his house with his friends while his parents went about their daily chores. When Selim had been gone for some time, Shilpee became anxious and, with the help of neighbours, started searching for him. Tragically, Selim was eventually found dead in the pond. No one knew exactly how he had drowned. The sudden death of the young boy was extremely painful for the parents.

Two years after Selim's death, a child day-care centre was established in his village. Sayed and Shilpee wasted no time in putting their other two sons, Mridul (aged 3) and Siam (aged 1), into the centre. At the cost of their son's life, the couple had realized the importance of keeping children in such a centre. The two boys now enjoy being at the day-care centre, and Sayed and Shilpee know they are safe while they are at work. Now the parents encourage other parents to send their children to the day-care centre too.

Day-care programme sustainability is a challenge, and inevitably will require commitment of partners from outside the community. But in the quest for sustainability, programme implementers should not overlook the value of committed champions such as Sayed and Shilpee who come from the community and who can become the most vocal proponents of the lifesaving value of this type of intervention.

2
Install barriers controlling access to water

Globally, the highest rates of drowning deaths occur among children aged 1–4 years, most of whom drown very close to home *(1). The Global report on drowning* identifies risk factors for child drowning as absent or inadequate supervision and barriers preventing access to water, and low hazard awareness *(1)*.

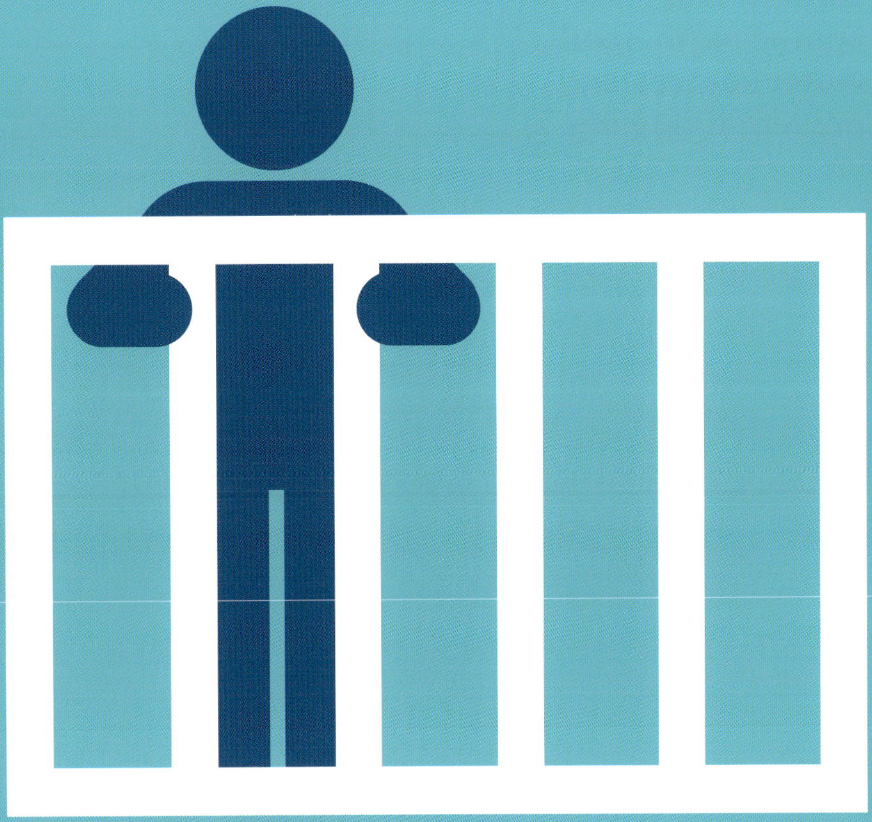

Benefits of installing barriers controlling access to water

Physical barriers can stop children coming into contact with open water sources and prevent drowning. Some high-income countries have done much to reduce childhood drowning using this strategy and there is potential to do the same in low- and middle-income countries.

In high-income countries most childhood drowning occurs in inadequately or unfenced swimming pools, and four-sided or isolation fencing with a self-closing and self-latching gate has been an effective prevention strategy *(1, 5)*. In Australia, drowning in farm dams is a major risk for young children, and steps have been taken to create safe play areas in order to reduce it *(6)*. In low- and middle-income countries, anecdotal evidence and studies of drowning indicate that natural bodies of water pose the greatest risk for child drowning. Covering or fencing-off open water may be impractical, especially in places with many nearby water bodies *(7)*. In these settings, installing doorway barriers in the home, using playpens, or fencing-off a safe play area in or around the family home can be a simple and affordable alternative, and help with supervision *(7, 8, 9)*. These options have been introduced and their effectiveness is being actively explored *(10, 11)*.

Physical barriers can stop children coming into contact with open water sources and prevent drowning.

Box 1: Potential standards for installing barriers controlling access to water for drowning prevention

- EN 12227:2010, Playpens for domestic use – safety requirements and test methods
- ASTM F406-13, Standard consumer safety specification for non-full-size baby cribs/play yards
- EN 1930:2011, Child use and care articles – safety barriers
- ASTM F1004-12, Standard consumer safety specification for expansion gates and expandable enclosures
- AS 1926.1-2012, Swimming pool safety – safety barriers for swimming pools
- European Standard/Europäische Norm (EN) https://www.cen.eu
- American Society for Testing and Materials (ASTM) http://www.astm.org
- Australian Standards (AS) standards http://www.standards.org.au

Installing barriers controlling access to water

Barriers controlling access to water are a strategy for child drowning prevention, but standards for such barriers do not exist in low- and middle-income countries. It is however possible to learn from high-income countries and adapt their standards (see Box 1).

Step one

Assess the situation in relation to barriers to water

See page 5

As part of your situational assessment, consider any existing water development and disaster risk reduction sector interventions that may impact community access or exposure to water.

Step two

Define target group/s

The target group will depend on the water hazard and the most appropriate barrier to protect against it; playpens may be appropriate for children aged 0–24 months, though if used improperly they can potentially increase drowning deaths; door barriers for children between 6 months and 4 years; pool fencing for children aged 6 months to 6 years; and barriers around wells for children aged 6 months to 6 years. Fencing around rural homes, including a child-proof gate latch, can prevent children wandering into waterholes, dams or irrigation channels.

Older children and adults can also have potentially dangerous access to water controlled by barriers, for example by covering open manholes and installing guardrails at or around dangerous water points such as waterfalls etc. There are some interventions in high-income countries that encourage or require the use of barriers around open bodies of water such as ponds in gardens or rural areas *(12)*.

Step three

Design and implement barrier interventions

The four main barrier interventions in the *Global report on drowning* are playpens, doorway barriers, pool fencing, and cistern, tank or well covering.

Playpens[6]

A playpen is a four-sided enclosed structure, usually with vertical slats or mesh sides and a base *(8, 9)*. It may be

6 Improperly used playpens may increase the risk of drowning deaths.

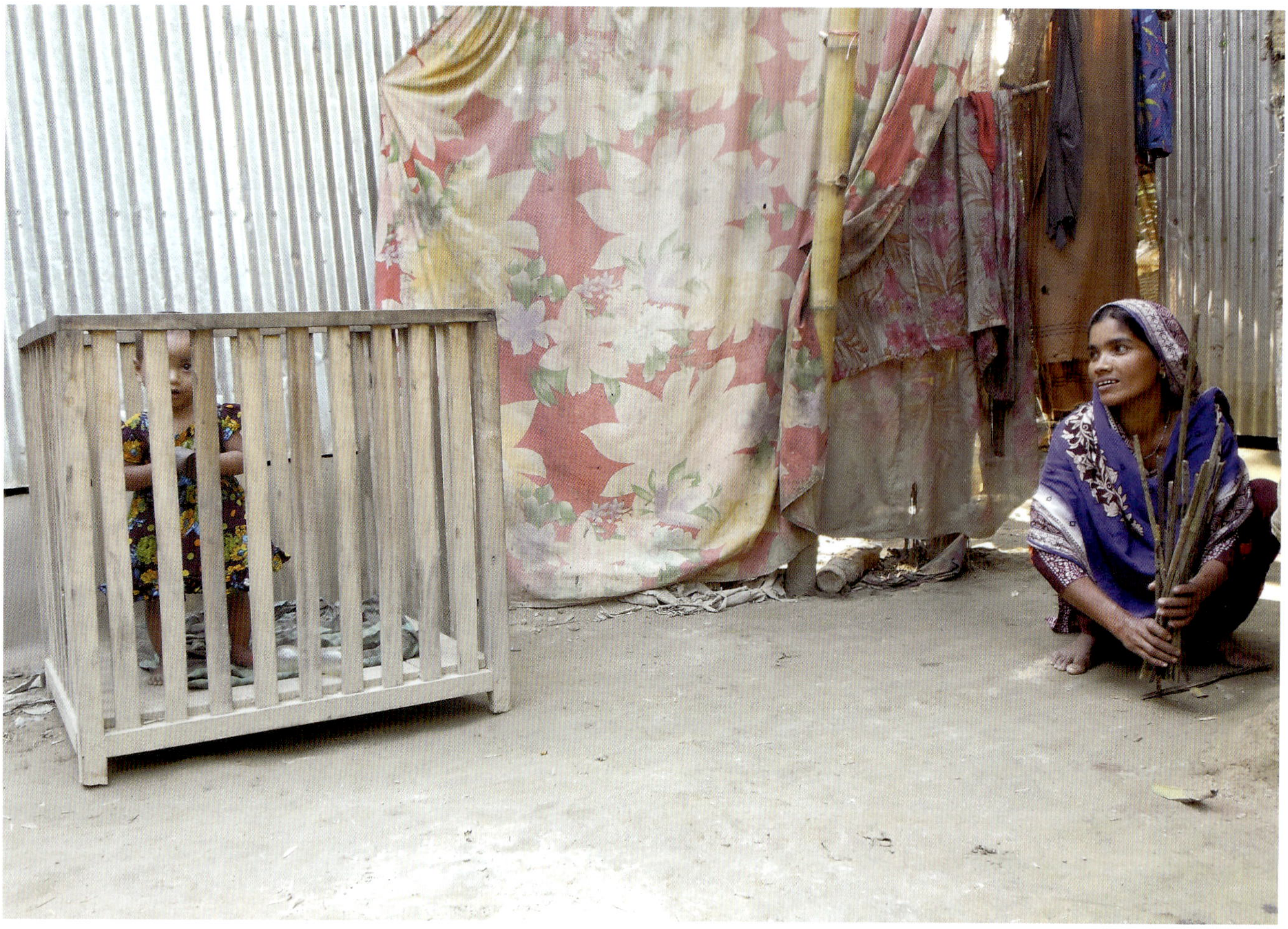

The four main interventions are playpens, doorway barriers, pool fencing, and cistern, tank or well covering.

handmade, procured locally or imported. It is important to ensure that playpen materials and design pose no injury or other health risks to children. When used as recommended, (see Box 2), playpens have been found to be very safe *(13)*. To date, drowning prevention programmes in low- and middle-income countries have used a wide variety of locally made or imported playpens and materials (including metal, wood, plastic, mesh and fabric *(8–10, 14)*.

Playpens designed and built locally should consider the typical house size and space available *(11)*. Bulky or heavy playpens may be underused if hard to move, while very light playpens may be unstable or unable to withstand a child kicking them. Playpen slats must be vertical, as horizontal ones can enable a child to climb out *(15)*. Slats must be no more than 60 mm apart *(16, 17)*.

The recommended minimum side-height for playpens is 0.5 m or 20 inches (and for cribs which are to sleep children, 0.66 m or 26 inches) *(14, 16)*. While most children aged up to 24 months cannot cross a 0.66 m high barrier, children aged 24 months to 4 years can easily climb barriers double that height *(18)*. Playpens are therefore considered to offer protection for children up to 2 years and carers must be advised on their safe use, including how to monitor the child's abilities to climb out (see Box 2).

Children mature rapidly and need to be continually monitored in terms of their physical abilities to potentially climb out of a playpen.

Box 2: Key messages for safe use of a playpen *(17, 19, 20)*

Playpens should not be considered a failsafe means of preventing harm, and if improperly used can increase the risk of drowning deaths. Children mature rapidly and need to be continually monitored in terms of their physical abilities to potentially climb out of a playpen. Similarly, children should not be left in playpens and unsupervised for long periods of time. Children left in playpens may cry and be removed from the playpens by siblings or another family member – if they are removed from the playpen they are clearly able to move around their environment and may drown. Caregivers using a playpen need to be aware of this risk.

- Place playpen in a safe location away from fire, heat sources or other hazards.
- Keep playpen away from cords, clothes lines, hanging ropes etc. as these can strangle children.
- Place playpen at ground level and on an even surface.
- Do not use if unstable or structurally unsound.
- Do not use if the child can climb out.
- Do not use if there are splits, cracks, or rough, sharp edges, corners or surfaces.
- Do not use if there are protrusions such as wing nuts or bolts that can strangle a child if clothing is caught.
- Do not use if there are missing slats.
- Do not use blankets, wraps, quilts or sheets when the child is in the playpen as these can increase suffocation risk.
- Playpen mattresses must be firm and tight fitting.
- Do not put large toys or boxes in the playpen as the child can use them to climb out.
- Toys and other items should not be tied at the corner or on the top of the playpen railing as these can strangle a child.
- Check the railing for holes and tears as children may bite the top railing during teething; discontinue use if these cannot be repaired.
- Never let children play with plastic wrapping or bags.
- Do not tie anything around a child's neck (threads, amulets, necklace, bibs, pacifiers etc.) in case the tied object gets caught on the playpen.
- Do not cover the playpen when the child is in it.

Doorway barriers

See page 23

Although there is no standard definition of a doorway barrier, in high-income countries commercially available safety barriers (sometimes called safety gates or baby gates) are used to prevent injuries among very small children around the house. Relevant standards are given in Box 1. Doorway barriers have been implemented in a range of countries to prevent drowning, including the Philippines *(21)* and Bangladesh *(10)*. All household members must ensure they have closed the barrier behind them – or better still, use a self-closing barrier. As with playpens, monitoring a child's ability to climb over the barrier applies, although it is worth noting that doorway barriers can be higher than playpens. Ensuring the child cannot open it is important and usually involves either a mechanism requiring strength greater than the child can apply or a complex mechanism (e.g. one requiring the user to simultaneously squeeze and lift).

Fencing around swimming pools

Legislation requiring isolation or four-sided pool fencing with self-closing or self-latching gates can reduce drowning among children in swimming pools *(5)*. Furthermore, increasing the height of the fence makes crossing the barrier more challenging – a 1.4–1.5 m high barrier is effective for children aged under 6 years *(15, 18)*. Barriers should be non-climbable, robust and regularly inspected for faults that may allow entry.

Covering wells, water containers and cisterns

Open wells, underground cisterns and containers holding water increase the risk of child drowning *(22)*. Covering and securing (or emptying) these water sources (such as turning a washing bucket upside down after use) can prevent drowning. A physical barrier around a well or cistern must be sturdy, sufficiently high to prevent children or adults from falling in, and designed so that young children cannot climb it. Another intervention to reduce people's need to access potentially hazardous water bodies could be installing underground plumbing, closed irrigation or a pump to safely draw water, although the impact of this on drowning has not been extensively studied.

⇩ Step four

Implement legislation to support interventions

As discussed, legislation requiring four-sided or isolation fencing with a self-closing or self-latching gate has increased the effectiveness of this intervention in some countries. However, for such legislation to be effective, all pools – old and new – must adhere to it *(9, 23)*. Stringent pool fencing may not be effective if compliance is low or enforcement is weak *(24, 25, 26)*. Pool-fencing legislation must therefore be

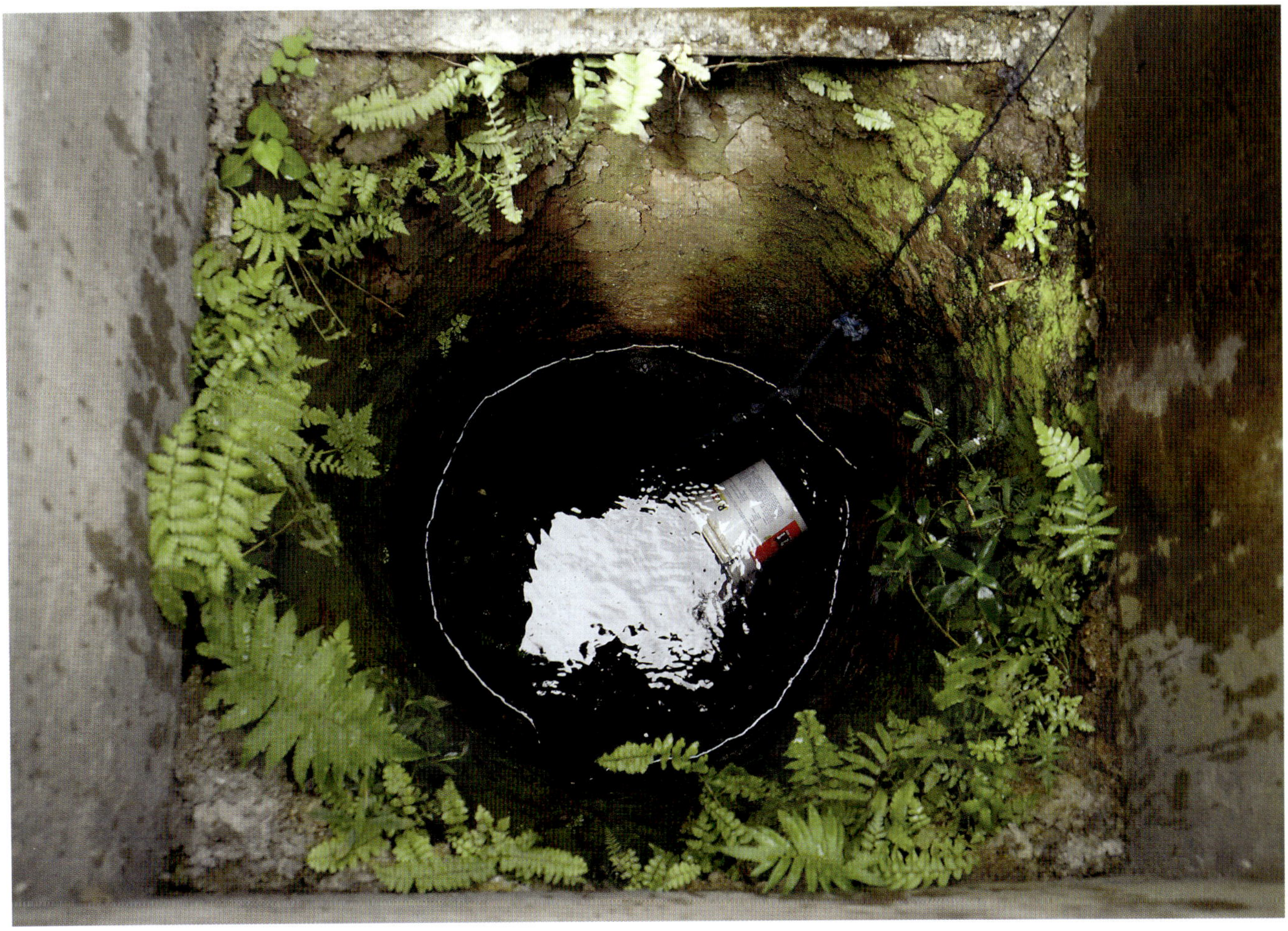

A physical barrier around a well or cistern must be sturdy, sufficiently high to prevent children or adults from falling in, and designed so that young children cannot climb it.

accompanied by active awareness-raising efforts directed at the community, and enforcement measures *(24, 25)*. Legislation on covering open wells and cisterns (or deactivating abandoned ones that can accumulate water) may also prevent drowning, although this is another area where research will help clarify potential impact.

⇩ Step five

Monitoring and evaluating interventions

While it is not possible to monitor the implementation of playpens, doorway barriers and covering of wells and water containers in individual homes (unless as part of a research study), monitoring and evaluation can focus on whether safe and appropriate messages are being disseminated, for example, on what sort of playpens should be provided and how they should be constructed; the availability of safe playpens and doorway barriers; and assessing the use of playpens and barriers when investigating drowning cases.

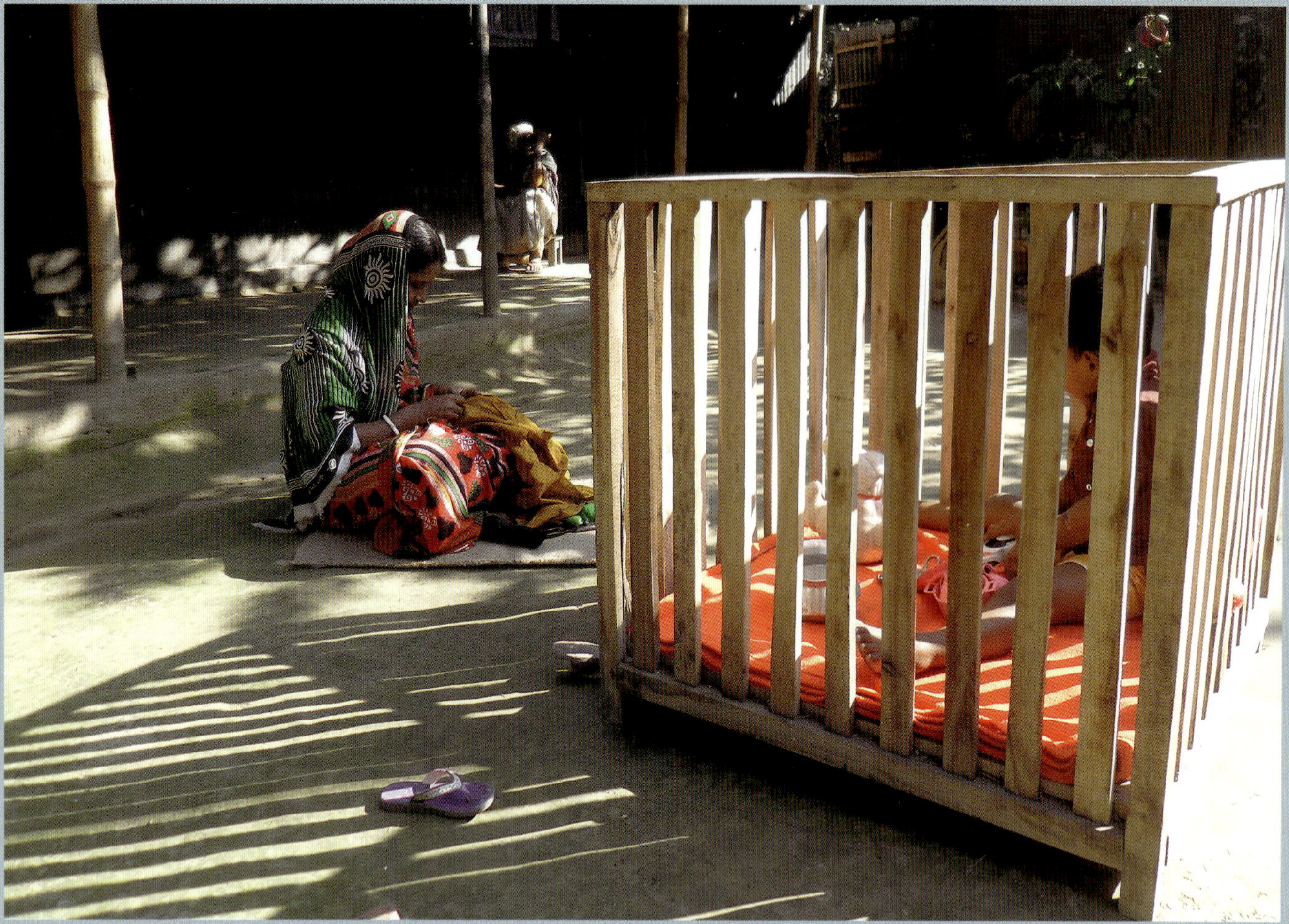

Case study

Implementing the use of playpens[7] and day care, Bangladesh

Saving of Lives from Drowning (SoLiD) is a large-scale implementation research study being conducted in seven sub-districts of Bangladesh to assess effectiveness and cost-effectiveness of two drowning prevention interventions – playpens and day care – among children aged under 4 years. About 75 000 children aged between 9–36 months are enrolled in the study. Enrolled children receive either a playpen or access to a day-care centre, or both. Two different types of locally manufactured playpens – wooden and plastic – are distributed. All enrolled children are followed up at regular intervals as part of a compliance assessment and to provide support and education to carers.

Preliminary findings indicate that both playpen and day-care interventions are acceptable to the community for child drowning prevention, and drowning incidence among children aged 0–4 years in the study area is three times lower than the historical rates *(8, 9)*.

7 Improperly used playpens may increase the risk of drowning deaths.

3

Teach school-age children (aged over 6 years) swimming and water safety skills

Drowning is a leading cause of child death in countries of all income levels, though low- and middle-income countries account for over 90% of child drowning globally *(27)*. This has led to increased interest in teaching swimming skills as a way to prevent drowning.

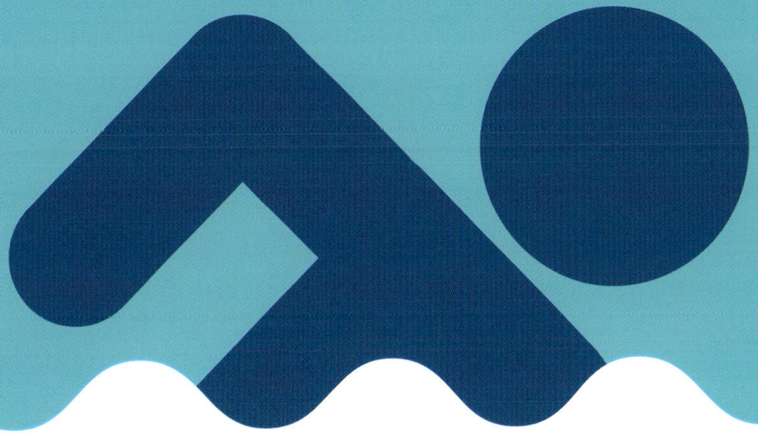

Globally, drowning rates are highest in early childhood and decrease rapidly in middle childhood. In low- and middle-income countries drowning rates further decrease in adolescence *(28)* but in many high-income countries they rise because of recreational drownings in places such as lakes and rivers. In low- and middle-income countries children drown in nearby water bodies during daily activities *(29)*. Drowning prevention in these different environments requires differing skills and proficiencies.

Perceived benefits of teaching swimming and water safety skills

Evidence that teaching children to swim protects them from drowning has only recently been established. A 2014 review of swimming and training curricula in high-income countries found little conclusive evidence of drowning reduction due to swimming *(30)*. However, the review found three case-control studies showing associations between receiving swimming lessons or naturally acquired swimming ability and decreased drowning *(31–33)*. It also found one trial, the SwimSafe Cohort Trial *(34)*, that showed an actual reduction in fatal drowning among school children in rural Bangladesh (see case study).

Schools are the preferred entry points for swim skills and water safety training.

Teaching a child to swim can be hazardous if appropriate safety measures are not in place. Recognizing this, high-income countries have developed formal programmes to teach children swimming that are often supported by government, reinforced by school curricula, certified by appropriate bodies, taught by trained and accredited instructors, evaluated for learning effectiveness and tested for safety. In general, participating children are aged 6 years or older, screened for risk (e.g. for epilepsy, asthma, disabilities) and taught in clean, clear, shallow water with highly visible boundaries. Swimming is taught as one component of a programme including water safety and safe rescue, and knowledge and attitudes to water.

See page 36 for Box 3 and Box 4

In low- and middle-income countries, conditions such as malnutrition, birth injury with physical and/or mental disability, asthma and epilepsy have high prevalence before the age of 6 years and are hard to screen for in these settings. This can put children aged under 6 years at risk of drowning during swimming lessons if they have such undetected conditions (see Box 3 on teaching children to swim in low- and middle-income settings and Box 4 on teaching high-risk children to swim). Preventing drowning among children aged under 6 years must therefore use other strategies such as barriers to water and capable supervision.

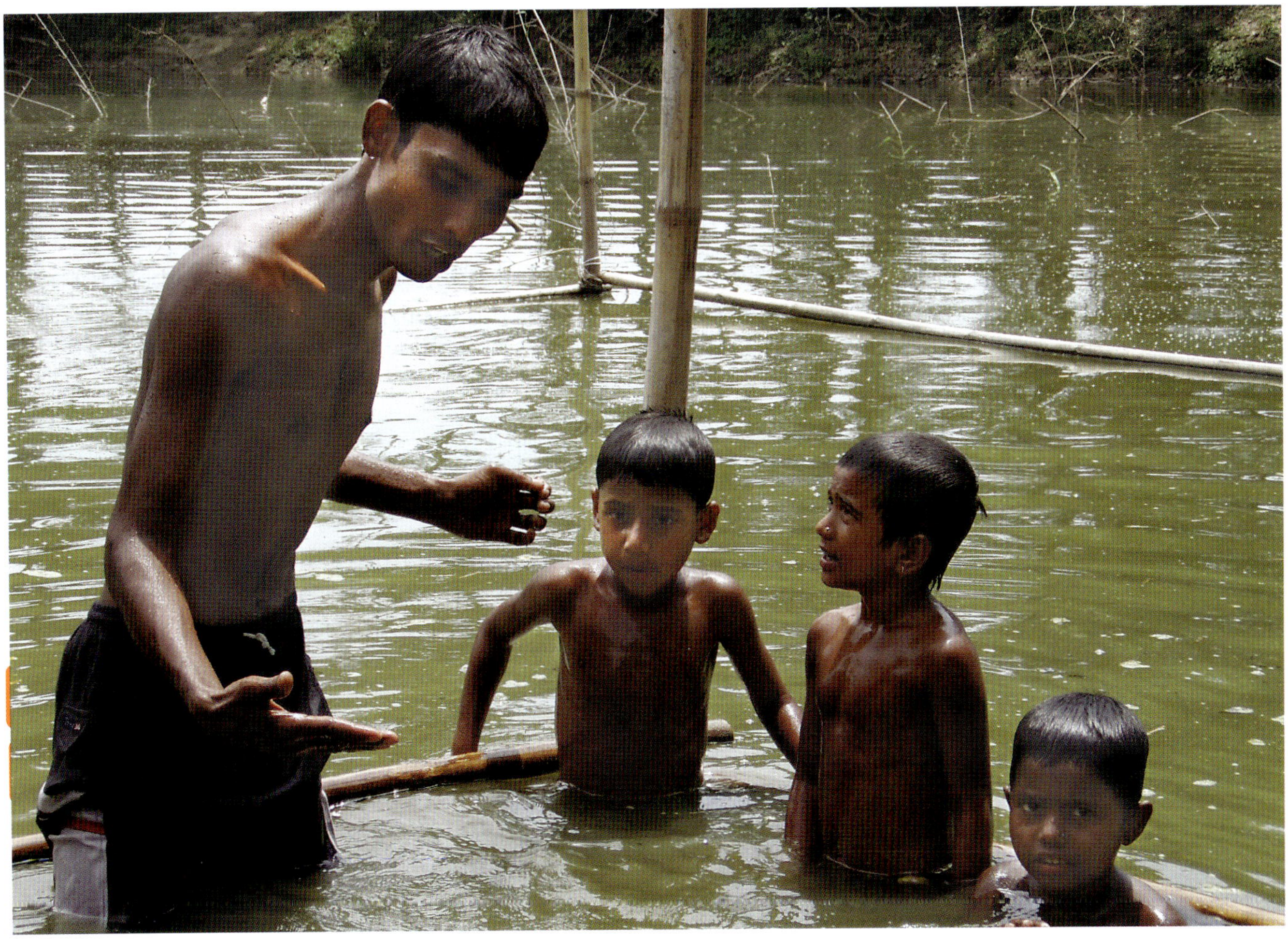

Implementing the teaching of swimming and water safety skills

⇩ Step one

Assess the swim skills and water safety situation

See page 5

Include schools as part of your situational assessment. Schools are the preferred entry points for swim skills and water safety training because they can provide training venues with teachers already experienced in classroom management and who have credibility with parents; on-site health staff; and (potentially) access to secure, access-controlled, fenced sites for pools (see Box 5 on benefits of school-based training in low- and middle-income countries).

See page 38

⇩ Step two

Define target group

The target group should be restricted to children aged 6 years or older who have been screened and found not to have underlying conditions that place them at increased risk.

Protocols relating to teaching children who are at increased risk are still being researched and defined; in the absence of these, school-based programmes that use medically trained

staff for screening, and with certified swim teachers using a curriculum designed for children at increased risk, are pre-requisites.

Risk management and teaching procedures to safely allow children under 6 years of age to participate in the SwimSafe curriculum are being tested at the time of writing. Evidence available to date from SwimSafe suggests that successful completion of training in the SwimSafe programme does not exceed 80% until 8 years of age.

⇩ Step three

Select training site

See page 38

Teaching swimming and water safety skills in a school setting has many advantages and provides the greatest measure of child protection (see Box 5). In settings with high levels of drowning, natural water bodies tend to be abundant. The SwimSafe programme itself was developed for use in different water bodies: in-ground pools, portable pools, ponds, reservoirs, lakes and beaches. All sites must be adapted for safety and risk management. Ponds and reservoirs require fenced, subsurface platforms to provide safe, uniform depths. Unbounded water bodies such as lakes also require subsurface platforms, as well as physical boundaries to ensure safe instructor-student separation is not exceeded. Beaches require floating boundaries to contain students, strategic site placement to avoid strong currents and other hazards, and attention to tidal conditions to ensure safe depth is not exceeded.

While microbial hazards can be an issue, especially in rural ponds, the major safety concern is poor water visibility – if a child has a seizure, falls or loses consciousness in cloudy water, they cannot be seen when submerged. Without clear water, risk management relies on screening out children at increased risk,[8] minimizing instructor distraction, ensuring the presence of safety monitors and maintaining small class sizes. Waterborne diseases may be an issue in some low- and middle-income countries. For example, schistosomiasis may be a significant barrier to implementing large-scale, fresh-water swimming programmes in Africa.

8 Unless, as mentioned in step 3, "Define target group", the programme is school-based, uses medically trained staff for screening, and certified swim teachers using a curriculum designed for children at increased risk.

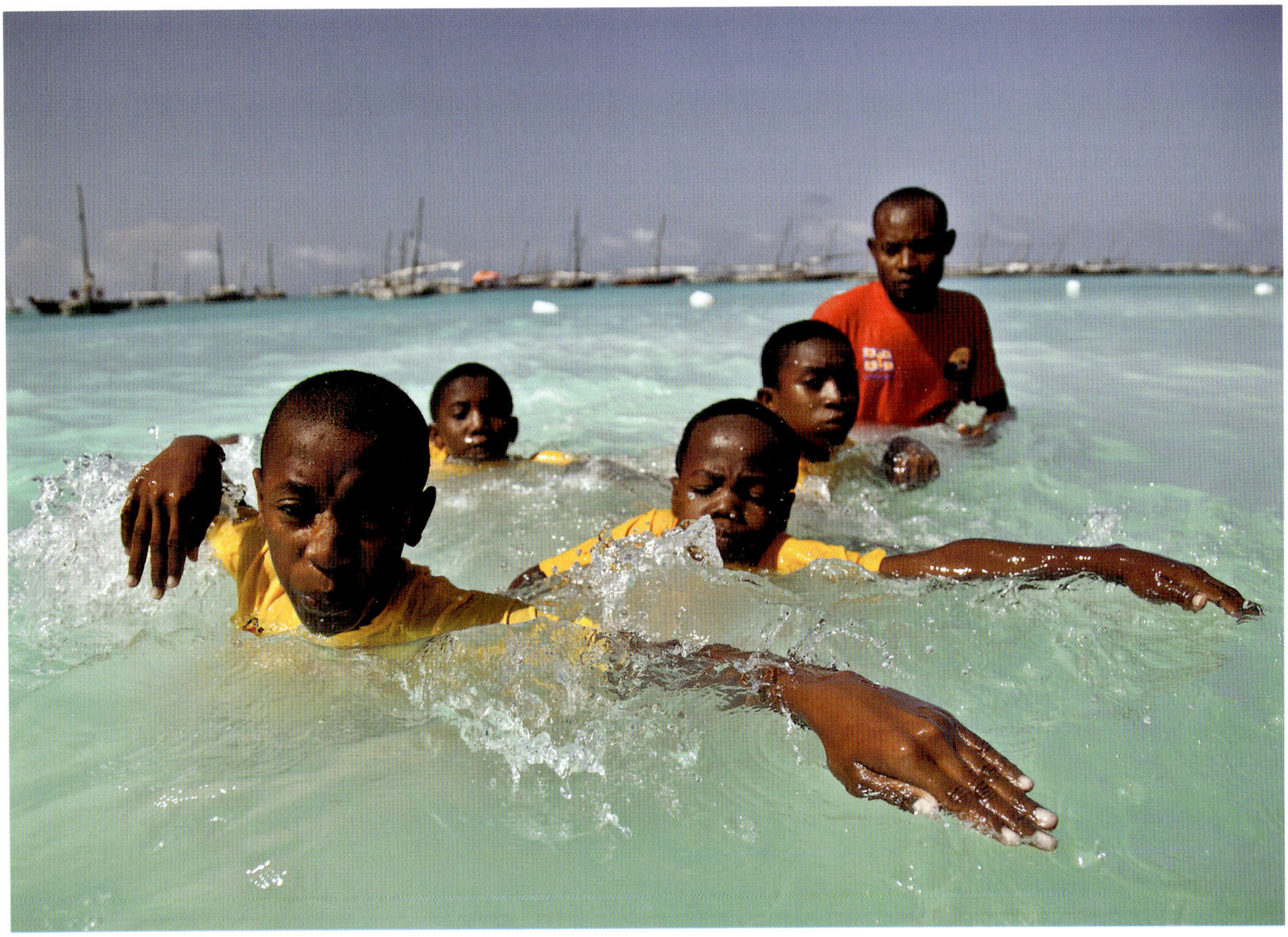

Swimming should be taught by adults who are native speakers; come from the local culture; and are trained and certified in both swim teaching and maintaining concentration and discipline with groups of children.

See page 38

⇩ Step four

Select and train instructors

Swimming should be taught by adults who are native speakers; come from the local culture; and are trained and certified in both swim teaching and maintaining concentration and discipline with groups of children – school teachers (ideally both male and female) are ideal. Swimsafe – the largest scale, best studied and evaluated programme – indicates that instructor-student ratios must not exceed 1:5 and may be lower (e.g. 1:1, 1:2, 1:3 or 1:4)[9] depending on supervision needs, particularly with children aged 6–9 years. In low- and middle-income countries where background checks are not robust or possible, community involvement in trainer selection may be useful for child protection. "Good character" references and ongoing monitoring from community leaders may be the only alternative to the background screening system used in high-income countries (see Box 6 on concerns around using volunteer teachers from high-income countries).

In Bangladesh, swimming instructors are selected from the community (approximately equal numbers of males and females); trained and certified in the SwimSafe curriculum,

9 The only place these ratios have been tested in non-school-based, rural programmes is as part of the SwimSafe programme.

cardiopulmonary resuscitation (CPR) and first aid; and trained to screen children for risk. In Thailand and Viet Nam, primary school teachers of both sexes are trained and certified in SwimSafe, CPR and first aid. Medical screening of students is done by the school nurse.

⇩ Step five

Engage parents

High-income countries already have protocols for teaching high-risk children to swim, but in low- and middle-income settings this is not the case.

Parents should participate in the assessment and screening of their children for swim teaching programmes, and attend information sessions. They should give informed consent and receive information about the programme – adapted for low literacy where appropriate. Information provided to parents should focus on water safety, the importance of active supervision and how to safely rescue a drowning child. Parental involvement is key in SwimSafe – often parental permission requires meeting cultural norms (e.g. same-sex instructors) and parents are the main source of knowledge for risk screening as they know most about current illnesses and previous episodes of seizures, asthma etc.

⇩ Step six

Monitor and evaluate

Process and output measures that should be recorded include personal information for all children participating (e.g. age, sex, name of child, name of parents, and addresses); the skill level obtained (e.g. dates of enrollment and date of graduation, failure or dropout); and any injuries or adverse events.

Box 3: Teaching children to swim in low- and middle-income settings

Based on current evidence, the following can be recommended for teaching children to swim in low- and middle-income settings:

- Enroll children aged 6 years and older.
- Obtain informed parental consent, a health and development history of the child and parental desires for culturally sensitive issues (e.g. swimming costumes, sex of instructor).
- Use trained health-care providers (if available) to screen children for conditions that increase risk; if not available, train and certify instructors in screening for these conditions.
- Use curricula that have been tested for safety and shown to provide (at a minimum) the ability for children to swim 25 metres and tread water for 30 seconds (for example the SwimSafe programme, see case study).
- Use local instructors certified in the curriculum, first aid and CPR.
- Use instructors who have training and experience in teaching and managing groups of children if available (e.g. school teachers); if not, provide training on child and teaching environment management.
- Teach in water bodies modified for safety and with clear water where possible.
- Require programmes to closely monitor teaching activities to ensure effective teaching and compliance with safety standards (e.g. correct student-teacher ratios).
- Implement active surveillance for injury and other adverse effects in participating children.
- Maintain records for all participating children, including personal information for the child and parents, and details on attendance, enrollment, graduation, failure or dropout, injury or other adverse outcome.

Box 4: Teaching high-risk children to swim

High-income countries already have protocols for teaching high-risk children to swim, but in low- and middle-income settings this is not the case (other than SwimSafe's research protocols). Some teaching venues in low- and middle-income countries are much riskier than others when teaching high-risk children to swim (i.e., rural, decentralized teaching programmes that are not school-based). The small evidence base that does exist suggests effective monitoring and supervision is very difficult and creates a risk that would contravene child protection norms. However, though evidence is lacking, school-based programmes could feasibly address most of the issues for high-risk children learning to swim. As such, a reasonable approach would be to implement and monitor closely the teaching of swim skills to high-risk children in school-based programmes.

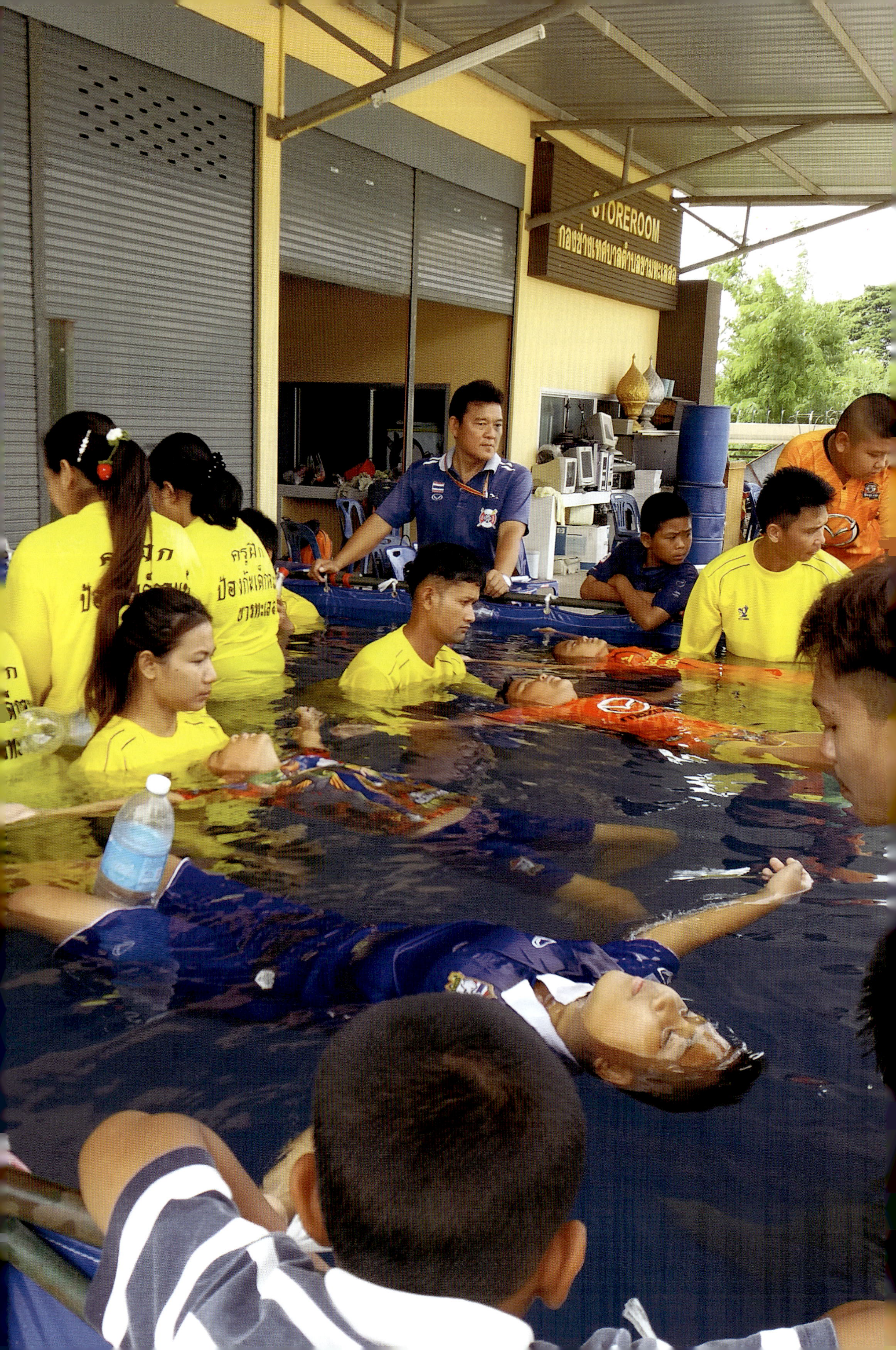
STOREROOM

Box 5: Benefits of school-based training in low- and middle-income countries

Where possible, school-based training provides the optimal combination of factors in low- and middle-income countries:

- Children of the same grade are of similar ages and physical development, making teaching more efficient.
- Teachers trained in classroom management are skilled in avoiding disruptions and distractions while teaching swimming.
- Schools maintain daily attendance registers to detect potential injuries and investigate dropouts.
- Meetings with parents for permission, risk-screening of the child and teaching water safety and supervision are easy to hold in schools.
- Many schools have a school nurse who can screen children for conditions that place them at risk, and other trained first-aid and CPR providers are often available from school health facilities.
- Many schools have security guards and provide increased security and fencing for pools.
- School grounds can be training sites if the school has a pool; portable pools can be used if not.
- Swimming classes before and after school, as well as during summer vacations, have been successful.

Box 6: Voluntourism (volunteer tourism): a word of caution

"Voluntourism" combines volunteering and tourism and refers to high-income country residents travelling to low- or middle-income countries to volunteer their skills, time and resources for short periods to local communities. However, there are concerns:

- The development value is debatable, with safety, community impacts, local job replacement and lack of cost-effectiveness and non-sustainability cited as disadvantages.
- Barriers and risks include lack of local language and cultural skills, and child protection issues.
- Many locations where children are at greatest drowning risk are far from tourism destinations.

Source: Wesby M. The help and harm of the 173 billion voluntourism industry. The Wilson Quarterly [website]. July 23, 2015.

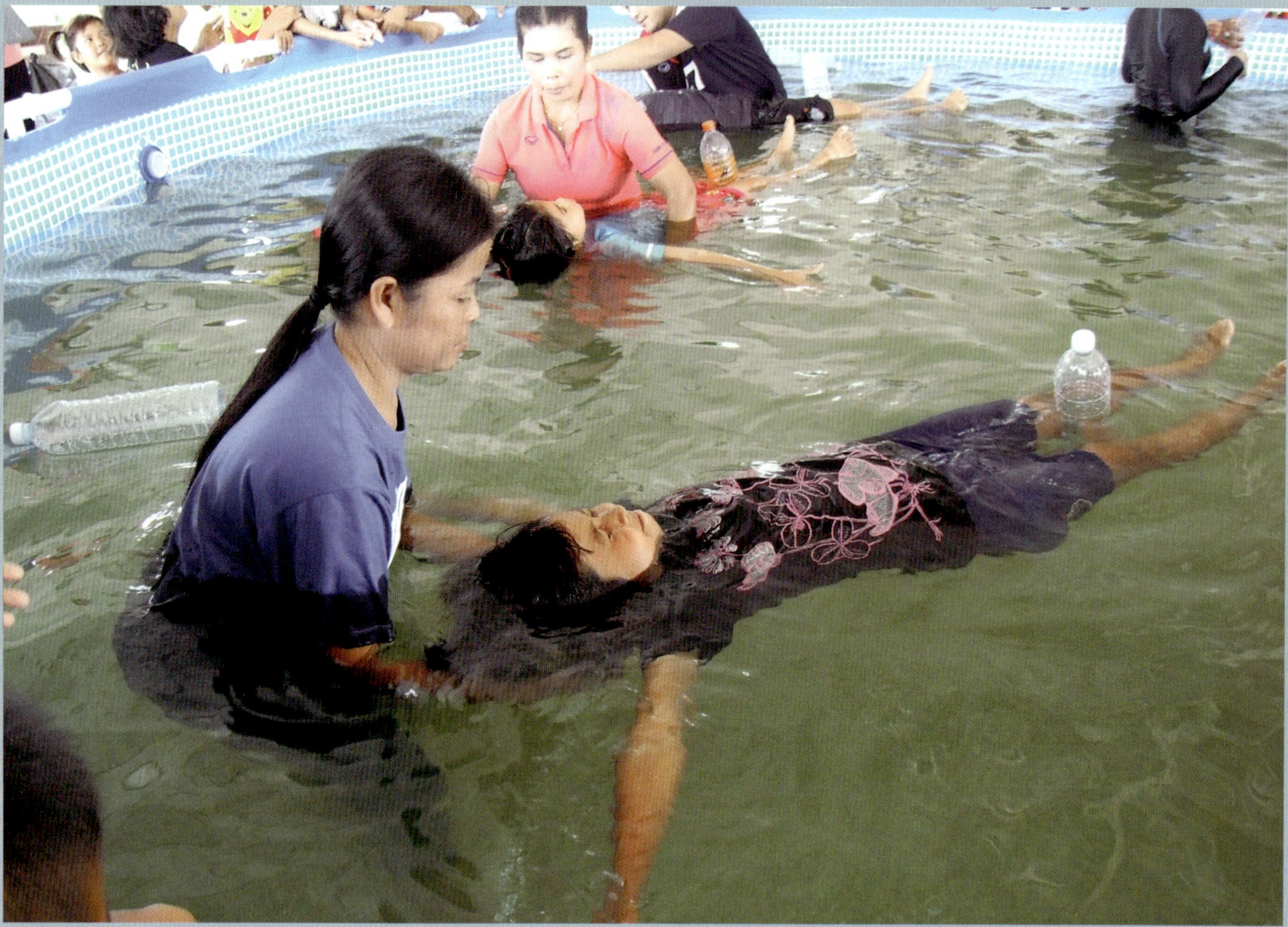

Case study
SwimSafe programme, Bangladesh, Thailand and Viet Nam

SwimSafe has been implemented in Bangladesh, Thailand and Viet Nam and provides practical information on teaching children to swim in low- and middle-income settings *(35)*. Since 2006, SwimSafe has taught over 525 000 children in a variety of teaching venues in these three countries. The experience underscores the risks and hazards present in low- and middle-income settings and shows the potential for swim teaching as a public health intervention. It provides robust evidence that children able to swim 25 metres and tread water for 30 seconds have lower fatal drowning rates in low- and middle-income country drowning environments. It shows most children aged under 6 years cannot achieve this skill level within the 21-lesson time frame. Importantly, a follow-up study has shown it does not lead to increased exposure or engaging in high-risk behaviours in the water *(36)*.

The experience in the three different countries has shown the importance of controlling factors relating to the site, parents, the child being taught, instructors, and the programme structure (see key steps for these factors). The SwimSafe curriculum teaches 18–22 basic swimming and water survival skills in up to 20 lessons. Teaching is done with a maximum ratio of 1 instructor to 5 students (there may be fewer students, depending on supervision needs, particularly with children aged 6–9 years).

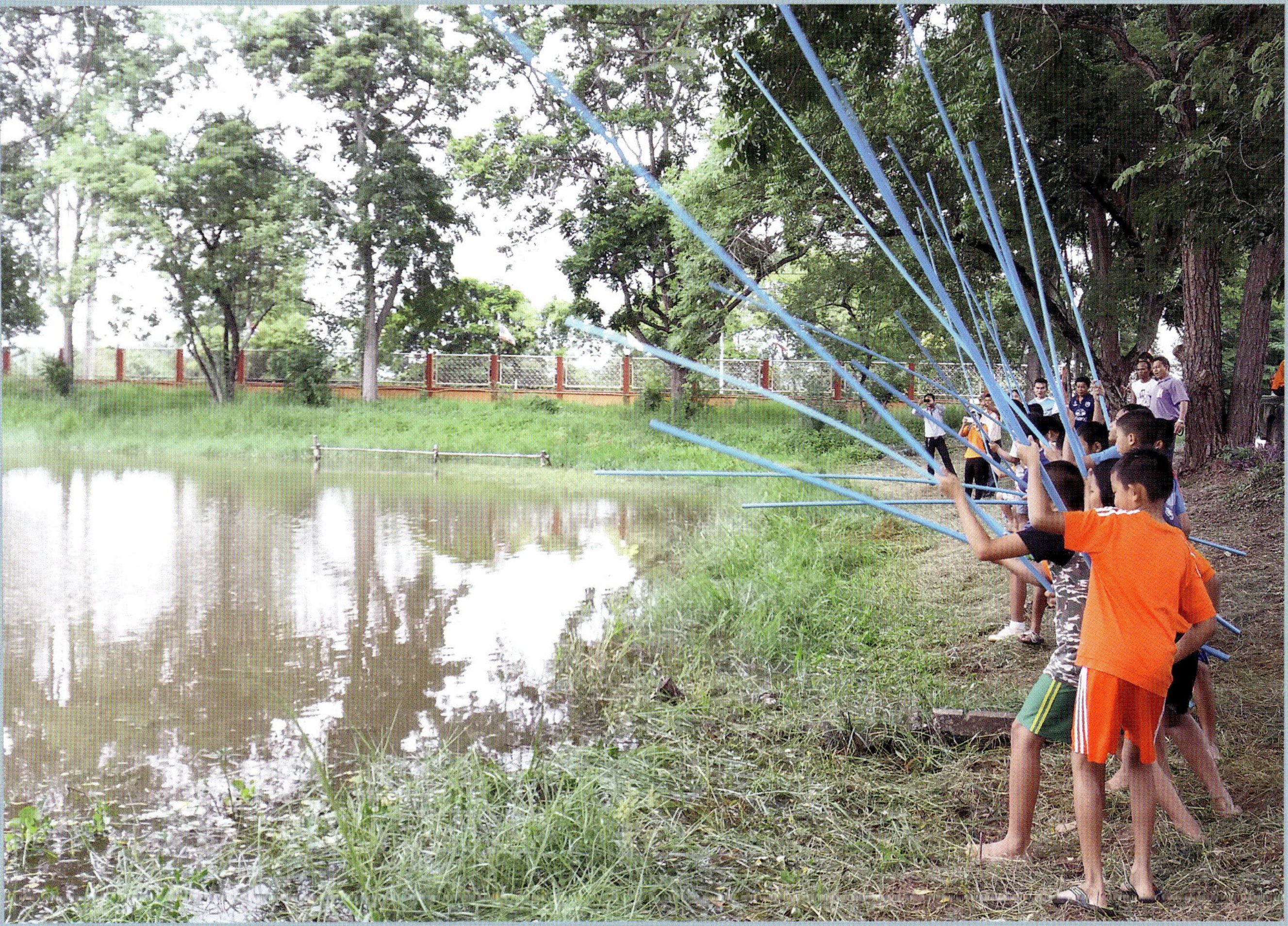

The skills/competencies taught are:

3 breathing skills:

- put face in water
- submerge and blow bubbles
- hold breath and exhale in submerged position

10 swimming skills:

- walk in the water
- walk with arm pulling
- float in the water with support
- float in the water without support
- kick by holding support
- push and glide without support
- push and glide with kick
- kick and pull with instructor or kickboard support
- kick, arm pull and breathing
- push, glide, kick and arm pull

2 survival competencies:

- swim 25 metres using any recognizable stroke
- float for 30 seconds

3 elementary rescue techniques:

- be rescued with a pole
- rescue others using pole and rope from edge of pond
- rescue others by throwing floating objects

Older children also learn safer "in-water rescue", as detailed study shows most rescues happen when children (both the drowning child and their peer rescuer) are already in the water *(37)*. See http://swimsafe.org for more information on the curriculum.

4

Build resilience and manage flood risks and other hazards

Flooding affects more people globally than any other natural hazard *(38)* and drowning has been identified as the most significant cause of flood deaths *(39–43)*, especially in Asia. In many regions of the world flood risk is expected to rise as a result of a mix of climate change *(44, 45)*, urban growth *(46, 47)* and environmental change *(48)*.

Benefits of building resilience and managing flood risks and other hazards

Despite the increasing frequency of flood disasters, in some regions deaths due to sudden floods and cyclones have nonetheless declined. This is thought to be the result of improvements in development conditions in low- and middle-income countries, and in early warning, disaster preparedness and response *(49)*. Building resilience to floods and related hazards enables communities to be safer from floodwaters (through levees, flood-resistant buildings, warning systems etc.) and to be prepared to reach shelter or safer ground if risk arises. Managing existing flood risk comprises a mix of structural (engineered) and non-structural approaches.

Build resilience and manage flood risks and other hazards

Managing existing flood risk comprises a mix of structural (engineered) and non-structural approaches.

The Sendai Framework for Disaster Risk Reduction 2015–2030 is a voluntary agreement that recognizes that while national government has the primary role in reducing disaster risk, responsibility should be shared with local government, the private sector and other stakeholders. It outlines global disaster risk reduction priorities, including those related to global flood risks *(50)*. In flood-prone communities, a risk management approach is necessary to minimize the risks posed by flooding, and includes the following steps.

⇩ Step one

Assess flood risk

To assess the scale and severity of flood risk, a risk assessment should be completed. This typically means undertaking detailed flood modelling and using outputs from this (such as inundation maps) to identify which parts of a community are at risk of flooding. Where detailed flood modelling is not available, historical information about flooding will help perform an initial assessment, including discussions with local people.

⇩ Step two

Select the most suitable flood risk management methods

Measures considered essential to any flood risk reduction approach include:

- Community education and engagement prior to flooding, ensuring residents are aware of flood risks and can take part in decisions on managing those risks. This could

Land-use planning is essential to the management of future flood risk, as the safest place to be during a flood is away from the affected area.

include community awareness about hazards in flood waters, currents, snakes, rapid water rise in storm-water drains, canyons, cycling or driving through flood waters etc. *(51)*.

- Establishing early warning systems using methods and technology appropriate to the setting. These must ensure accurate prediction and rapid dissemination to communities so they understand when and where flooding will occur and have time to evacuate to safety.
- Developing disaster response and recovery plans for floods where flooding risk is present, including arrangements for evacuation (where necessary). These plans should be drawn up with community involvement and aim to ensure adequate capacity to help communities respond to, and recover from, disasters. Plans should be regularly tested – community involvement is essential to this *(52, 53)*.
- Land-use planning is essential to the management of future flood risk, as the safest place to be during a flood is away from the affected area. Unrestricted development in at-risk areas results in life-threatening risks to safety, significant financial costs and community disruption *(54)*. Therefore land-use planning should ensure:
  - controls to limit worsening the flood risk by further development in at-risk areas *(55)*, and ensure all development is compatible with the nature of local flooding *(55)*;
  - complete evacuation of communities is possible in worst-case scenarios. This requires a warning system allowing enough time for residents to leave at-risk areas.
- Where practical, consideration should be given to the relocation of communities or properties, in particular after flood events, when re-development of flood-prone land is being considered.

Structural measures to mitigate the impacts of flooding must be considered in the context of specific flood-risk environments and include:

- constructing "hard" flood defences such as levees (banks) or coastal barriers to prevent flooding up to certain levels;
- raising the habitable floor level of existing properties and using flood-resistant building techniques;
- constructing shelters to enable people to evacuate to higher floors;
- constructing flood mitigation dams or basins to absorb floodwaters;
- urban stormwater management;

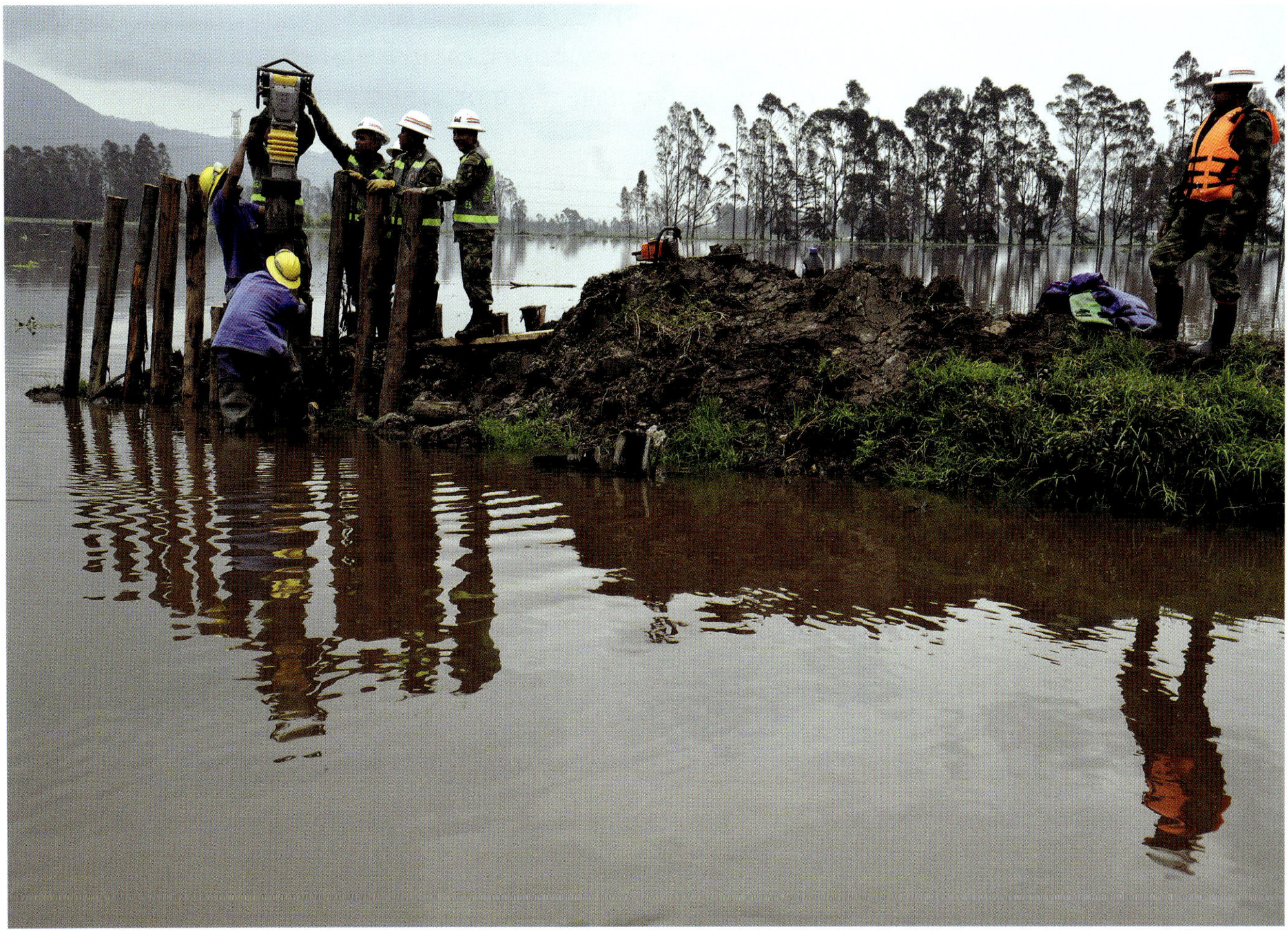

Flood defences require ongoing maintenance to ensure their strength and effectiveness.

- restoration of floodplains and vegetation to reduce run-off;
- channels to direct flood waters away from at-risk communities.

Flood defences such as these require ongoing maintenance to ensure their strength and effectiveness. A disadvantage of flood defences is that they may encourage further urban growth in protected areas *(38)*. Development behind defences should be managed carefully to avoid the intensification of flood risk that can happen during a severe flood that exceeds defence capacity. Dam construction must be linked to a robust dam safety programme to minimize the possibility of dam failure, or sudden releases of large volumes of water.

In the context of coastal flood risk management, promising alternatives or additions to "hard" flood defences are ecosystem-based approaches such as mangrove forests, wetlands and sand nourishment *(56, 57)*. There is mounting evidence that such approaches provide some protection through their ability to absorb the impact of waves *(57–59)* or buffer winds *(58)*. Some evidence exists that restoring floodplain forests can reduce river flooding *(60)*.

⇩ Step three

Develop and implement a flood risk management plan

At a local level, once appropriate approaches have been selected they should be shaped into a plan of action, prioritized, funded, monitored and evaluated. Overall, governance is of critical importance to the effective management of flood risk. Clear accountabilities, vision, plans, capability, guidance and coordination within and across all agencies and stakeholders are necessary to achieve effective results *(50)*. Key accountabilities of government agencies should be written into law. The plan should also include strategies around how life can return to normal after a flood, for example how and when schools and shops can re-open, or people can return to work, etc.

Flood risk management plans should be monitored and strategies should be regularly evaluated to test their effectiveness both before and after flood events.

⇩ Step four

Ensure drowning prevention is integrated with existing disaster risk reduction programmes

Communities at risk of flooding and coastal inundation may also have high rates of drowning in everyday life due to their proximity to water. The overlapping nature of drowning prevention interventions and those designed to build disaster resilience has yet to be fully explored but initial analysis suggests these communities can benefit from additional awareness-raising of the risks posed by water, and how to safely rescue people, etc.

⇩ Step five

Monitor and evaluate

Process measures that can be monitored include: presence or absence of flood risk management plans; establishment of entities at national, subnational and local levels to implement plans; frequency of meetings and activities such as scenario rehearsals; and establishment of things such as depots for pre-positioning of logistical supplies and communication campaigns to keep at-risk populations informed, etc. The implementation of flood risk management plans should be monitored, and strategies should be regularly evaluated to test their effectiveness both before and after flood events. The plan should be viewed as a living document with learnings incorporated to continually improve strategies.

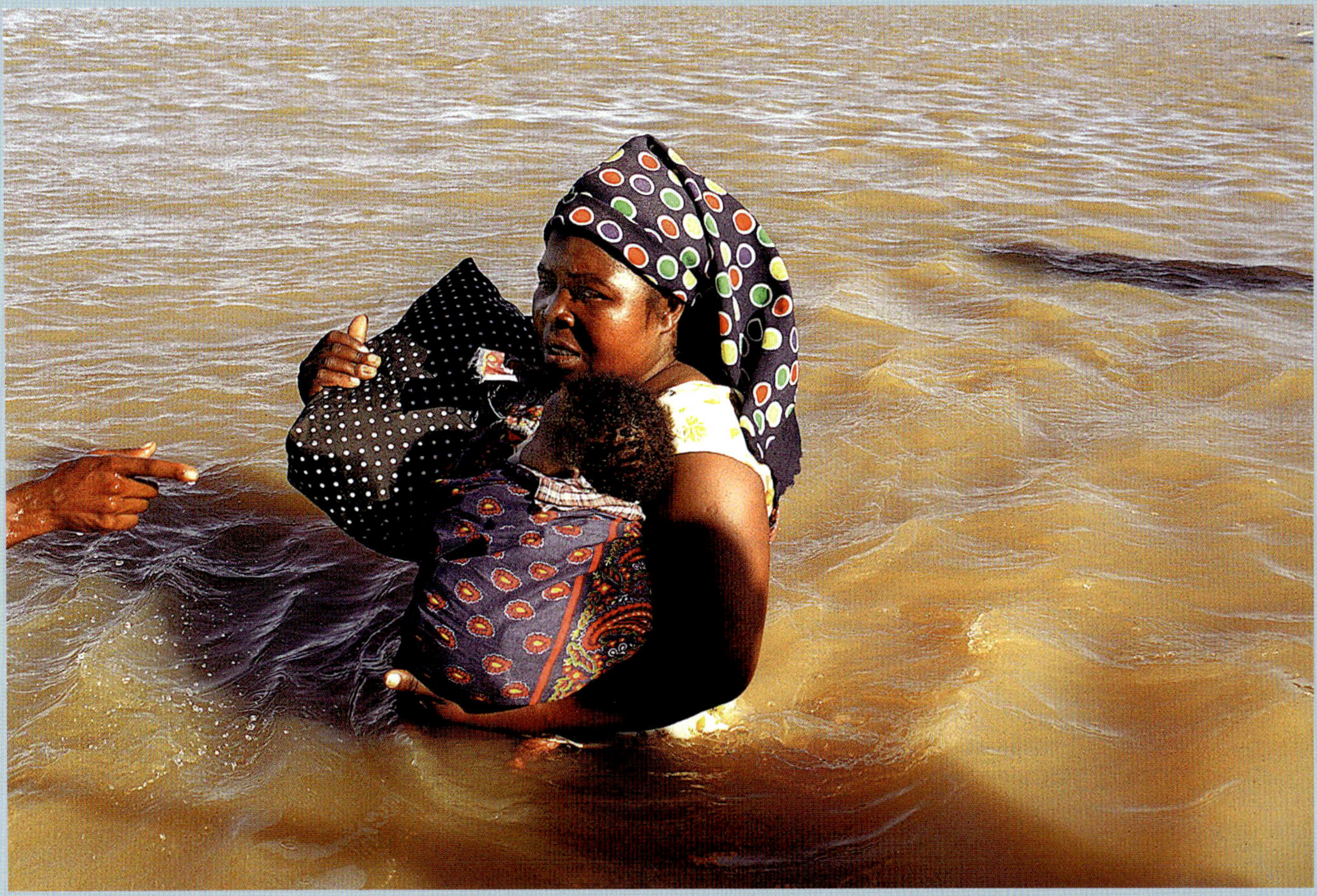

Case study
The impact of improved disaster risk response and management, Mozambique

In 2000, catastrophic floods in Mozambique killed over 700 people and left more than half a million people homeless. Overall, more than 4.5 million people were affected.

After the floods, the government took a range of measures to improve the effectiveness of the country's disaster risk management, including an Action Plan for the Reduction of Absolute Poverty, and a Master Plan which provides a comprehensive strategy for dealing with Mozambique's vulnerability to natural disasters. After the 2000 floods, a large resettlement programme for communities affected by the floods was initiated, with about 59 000 families resettled (though a lack of funds for improved livelihoods reduced the success of this programme). In addition, the Severe Weather Forecasting Demonstration Project got underway, which contributed to forecasts and warnings related to Cyclone Favio in February 2007.

In 2005 and 2006 the German Agency for Technical Cooperation developed a simple but effective early warning system along Mozambique's River Búzi, adapted to the specific needs of the people. Village officials receive daily rain and water level readings from strategic points along the river – if rain is particularly heavy or the river reaches critical levels, this information is passed on by radio, and blue, yellow or red flags are raised depending on the flood alert level.

Seven years after the catastrophic floods of 2000, similar flooding occurred in Mozambique, but the country was better prepared. While no loss of life is ever acceptable, the toll was nonetheless much lower than in 2000, with 29 people killed, 285 000 affected, and approximately 140 000 displaced. This reveals that developing effective and well-functioning systems of hydrological monitoring and early warning systems at a local, regional and national level is key to disaster risk management and realistic flood warnings.

Source: *(61)*

5

Train bystanders in safe rescue and resuscitation

Rescue and resuscitation have limited impact on reducing drowning mortality and morbidity (resources are more cost-effective when applied to drowning prevention *(62)*) but bystander rescue and resuscitation can nevertheless make the difference between life and death in individual drowning situations.

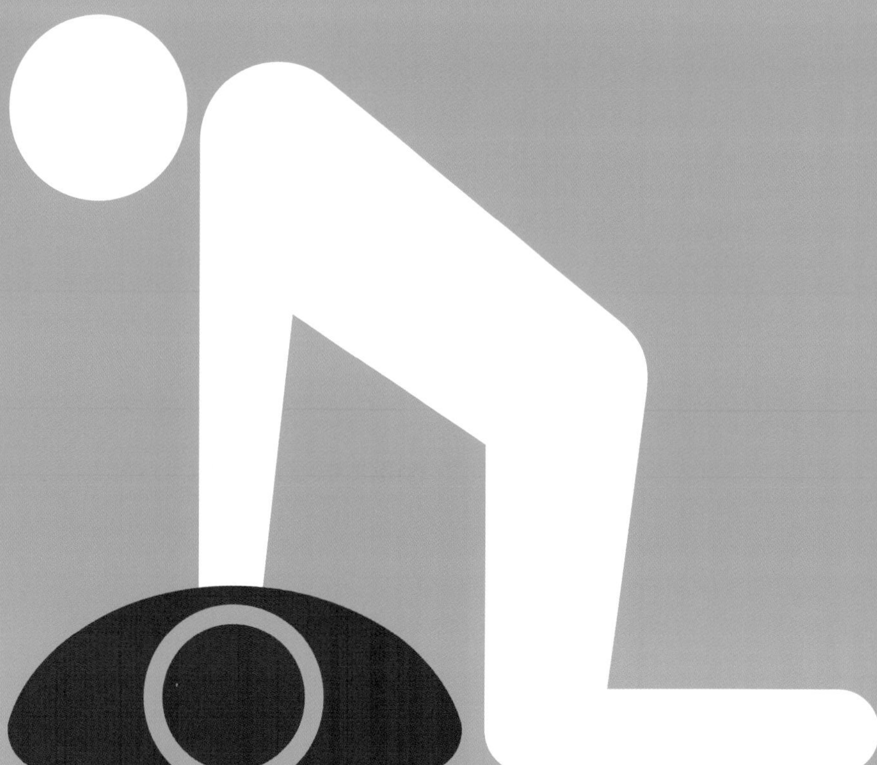

More qualitative and quantitative research is needed to improve understanding of the best way to train bystanders in safe rescue and resuscitation than is currently available. Many certified training programmes exist in high-income settings, but this guide focuses more on the best-known approaches to rescue or resuscitation training programmes in limited-resource settings, and on ensuring these programmes meet local learners' specific needs.

Benefits of training bystanders in safe rescue and resuscitation

Untrained people tend to help others in danger, even in extreme circumstances, and can place themselves at risk of drowning *(63, 64)*. Training allows people to act more safely when performing a rescue. Rescuers of drowning children are frequently other children;[10] this means interventions to train bystanders in safe rescue and resuscitation must consider carefully at what age such programmes can successfully train children. The age at which a child can start learning safe rescue and resuscitation techniques depends on physical ability. There is a general consensus that most children are physically able by the age of 12 years, and ongoing research suggests that in some instances such learning could happen earlier *(65)*.

Training bystanders in safe rescue and resuscitation

⇩ Step one

Assess the safe rescue and resuscitation situation

See page 5

Fact-finding and checking assumptions made during programme planning are critical to ensure a good fit to the local situation. Key concepts are that training needs to be adapted to the type of local water bodies, and that resuscitation protocols must also be suitable for the local culture as well as conform with established national protocols *(66–68)*. In addition to the discussion provided in the Situational assessment, Table 2 provides more detail on various elements to consider when establishing safe rescue and resuscitation training, including the lowest age at which children can start to learn these skills *(33, 37)*.

10 Data from Bangladesh show that the mean age of a person finding a drowning victim is twice the age of the drowning victim *(33, 37)*. Mean drowning mortality age in rural Bangladesh is 3.7 years, so CPR training for children aged 7–12 years is being trialled in the Bangladesh Anchal and SwimSafe (BASS) project, with Phase 1.5 results encouraging.

Table 2: Elements to consider in a situational assessment to prepare rescue and resuscitation training

Element	Examples
Culture	Gender, age, ethnicity, religion, beliefs, historical events, local policing
Partners	Local: swimming clubs, Red Cross, boy scouts, sea scouts, youth organizations, firefighters, prominent religious or political leaders, drowning casualties, their families and rescuers Tertiary physical education training institutions National: foundations, government, branches of international organizations
Water risk factors	Water body (e.g. river, lake, ocean, well, ponds or other high-risk areas), wave types, water depth, currents, temperature
Techniques	Understanding why traditional rescue and resuscitation techniques are important for the community (including those known to be ineffective or dangerous)
Target groups	Easily accessible: school children (aged 12 years, or possibly younger depending on circumstances), swimming class pupils, owners of and visitors to water leisure locations High risk: children who travel to school by boat or cross dangerous water, passengers of unsafe ferry boats, fishermen, cliff and lobster divers, detention and refugee centre populations, service personnel (police, army) High impact: parents, teachers, community leaders, health professionals, vessel operators (see Set and enforce safe boating regulations)
Students' level of knowledge	Knowledge of aquatics, human physiology, first aid, language; skills in swimming, self-rescue; medical conditions
Teachers	Use of the "train-the-trainer" model; being aware of the potential problems of using teachers from other countries (see Teach school-aged children swimming and water safety skills)
Local health system	Training should be tailored to the resources and equipment available

See page 54

See page 30

⇩ Step two

Select and train trainers

Gender, ethnicity, social background, availability and the empowerment of disadvantaged groups play a role in selecting local trainers. Once recruited and trained, trainers can benefit from periodic trainer re-certification, events to create a community among trainers and a sustainable funding programme. A local course director adds to programme sustainability *(69, 70)*. These measures can help retain trainers and prevent them leaving programmes to start their own teaching enterprise without feeding back on the quality, safety and content of those programmes.

See page 30

If needed, "train the trainer" approaches can be used to rapidly increase the number of trainers. These may require visiting trainers (appropriate to the local context) or be based around certified trainers from the host setting (see Teach school-aged children basic swim skills). If using visiting trainers, emphasis should be placed on tailoring teaching to local languages and needs (including using an interpreter to avoid translation errors), as well as working towards the gradual handover of all responsibilities to local counterparts.

⇩ Step three

Develop training methodology for trainers and students

Alongside traditional lecturing, other small-group teaching methods should be considered (e.g. songs, role-plays, quizzes and self-learning). Visual information, especially when referring to recognizable local settings, is often more effective than written information. Interactive learning creates better understanding than passive class attendance. In many cultures it is regarded as impolite to question the teacher or admit that something is not understood, so discussing pre-course questions is a good way to catalyse learner interaction and enhance training effectiveness.

The training setting should be realistic and use local material. One type of training setting simultaneously rotates trainers between 2–7 stations, with 4–6 students trained in one single skill over a set period of time. Performance of these skills is subsequently improved during scenario-simulation training. Regular breaks should be planned for feedback and reflection.

⇩ Step four

Develop course content

See page 54

Courses should ideally comprise more than half (and preferably three quarters) practical rather than theoretical content, and be concise, simple, practical and adapted to local conditions. Evidence-based and regularly updated, course content on rescue is available from several international and national organizations, commercial bodies and books *(71–75)* (see Set and enforce safe boating regulations for more on search and rescue).

Potential bystander rescuers should be trained using basic techniques that are easy to remember and safe to perform. Rescue training should emphasize rescuers' safety and safe use of rescue equipment. Training starts with simple, locally sourced rescue equipment (such as plastic containers) and progresses to more specialist (and therefore less readily available) equipment.

Practical training for resuscitation skills should focus on basic technical skills: ventilation (rate, time, volume) and chest compressions (rate, depth, hands-off time). Immediate mouth-to-mouth ventilation is critical in drowning. At the time of writing, guidelines developed by the European Resuscitation Council (ERC) are the most extensive and detailed, and therefore offer the best basis upon which to create locally adapted resuscitation content *(76)*. Resuscitation content should take into account the local health system, since the training should cover use of locally available equipment.

Non-technical skills (communication, leadership, situational awareness, feedback and the use of communication technology) are an important part of training. Other issues that need addressing may include gender and socio-economic status (for example men are not always allowed to touch women, and certain social or ethnic groups avoid contact); responsibility of transporting a drowning casualty to a hospital and potentially being asked to pay for the treatment; incorrect resuscitation techniques and unfounded fears of acquiring HIV or TB during mouth-to-mouth ventilation. Compression-only CPR is not appropriate after drowning and this point should be made clear.

An ethical dilemma is whether cardiac resuscitation should be taught when there is no ambulance system, local nurse, doctor or hospital to provide further treatment *(77)*. Survivors of successful mouth-to-mouth ventilation will generally not need further treatment, although 8 hours' clinical observation is advised *(78)*. Teaching only mouth-to-mouth ventilation may be considered in some settings where there is no further care available.

⇩ Step five

Develop training materials

Training materials must reflect the context of the local setting and be developed early in the preparation phase. They may include manuals, flip-charts, graphics, slides, checklists, flow-charts, mnemonics, DVDs, videos and long-distance learning via smart phone or Internet (e.g. Massive Open Online Courses). Blended learning – combining diverse learning methods and educational material – is often the most practical solution.

Potential bystander rescuers should be trained using basic techniques that are easy to remember and safe to perform.

Sophisticated training equipment such as mannequins or projectors is expensive, requires maintenance and does not always function well in hot, humid and bright environments. Lower tech training mannequins can be an excellent resource, along with low-cost equipment when training only includes mouth-to-mouth ventilation. Smart phones are increasingly available even in the poorest and most remote locations, and may be useful for providing video feedback.

⇩ Step six

Run refresher training

The retention time of resuscitation techniques is approximately 3–12 months in learners who have not used the skills in a real situation *(79)*. Refresher training is considered necessary and should be hands-on, including cognitive and practical skills. Posters, short videos and interactive lectures increase retention *(80)*. Instructors are advised to keep a log of all rescues or resuscitations performed by their students and provide feedback when a student has performed a rescue or resuscitation.

⇩ Step seven

Monitor and evaluate

Evaluation could encompass data to determine the reach and scale of the intervention (e.g. number of people trained, proportion of trained individuals receiving refresher training within a set period), as well as evaluation to determine the impact of training (e.g. records of where training has been put into action and outcome of that event). See Monitoring and evaluation.

See page 11

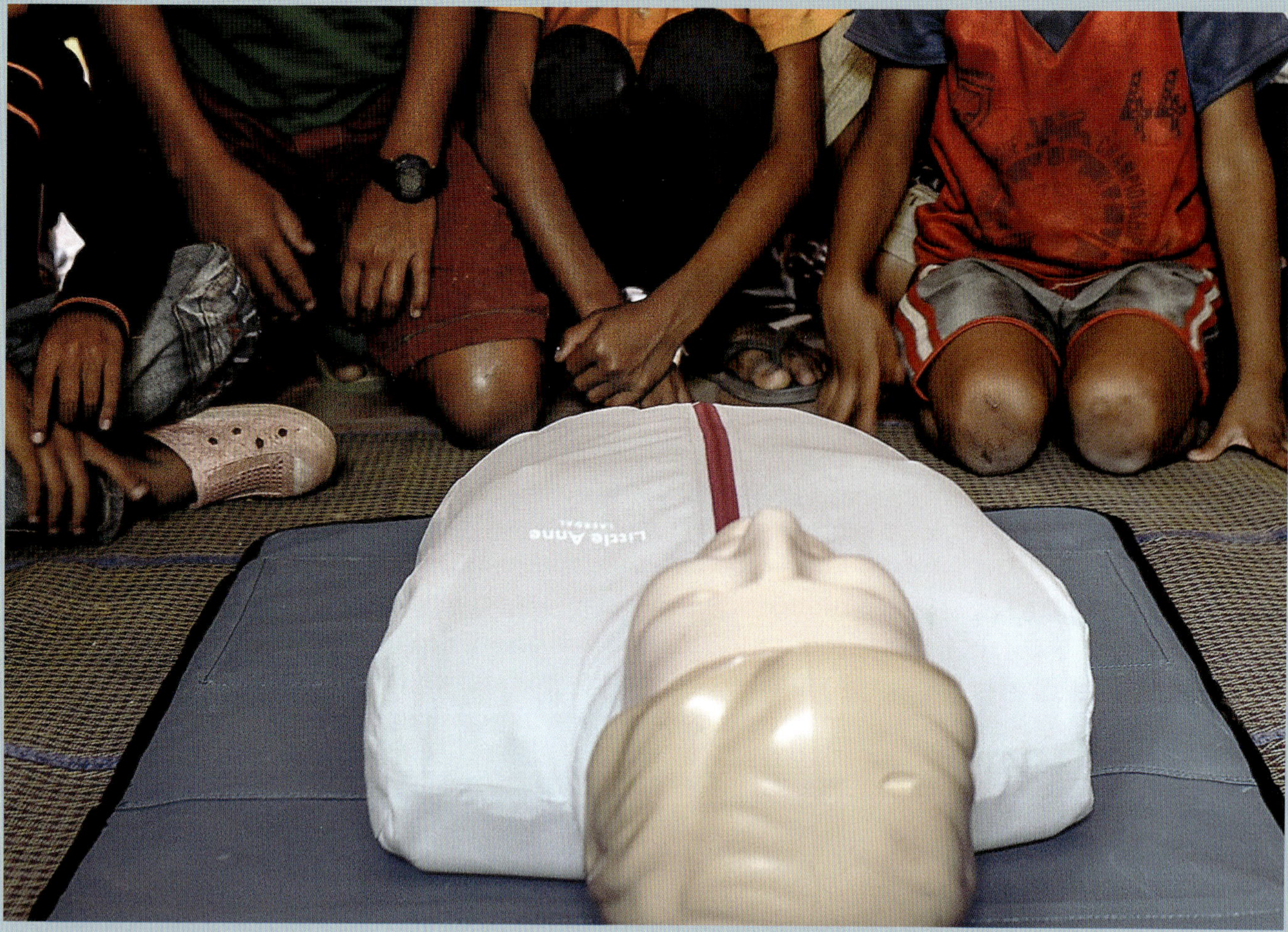

Case study
Developing safe rescue, Lesotho

Lesotho has no natural lakes and very few large rivers, so there is no tradition of swimming. Very few older people can swim, and parents often – unsuccessfully – forbid their children to swim too. In recent years, many small dams have been built in villages to stop soil erosion, and the country currently has two large lakes for hydro-electricity. Many children drown while playing.

The Royal Lesotho Lifesaving Association began by visiting locations during weekends where there was a swimming pool available, and invited nearby schools to send students who can swim. All students needed to be able to swim two lengths of the pool to prove swimming ability. On the first day of the course, students received training in rescue and resuscitation skills, and on the second day were assessed and – if successful – were awarded a basic certificate. Basic certificate teaching includes resuscitation and rescue by reaching, throwing, wading and swimming with an aid, assuming that the casualty is not too far from the shore. It is based on the Commonwealth levels 1, 2 and 3.

Those awarded a basic certificate were eligible to train for an intermediate certificate (roughly corresponding to Commonwealth level 4) which includes training in skills such as throwing a rope (overhand) while standing in water, or towing a casualty with a stick or with clothing. The final stage is the bronze medallion, and those who pass this can go on to become instructors themselves.

Since 2011, the Royal Lesotho Lifesaving Association has issued about 480 certificates, most of which have been at the basic level. Students who have been certified have come from 48 different schools or clubs. Data on impact are hard to obtain as not every drowning case or successful rescue are reported to police.

6

Set and enforce safe boating, shipping and ferry regulations

Making water transport safer for large and small vessels[11] requires both regulatory and educational interventions, which in turn depend on other behaviour-change initiatives such as training crew, generating a safety culture, and raising public awareness. Safety experts view regulation and enforcement and developing a safety culture as potentially the most effective measures to improve the safety of large vessels. They may be critical for improving safety on small vessels too.

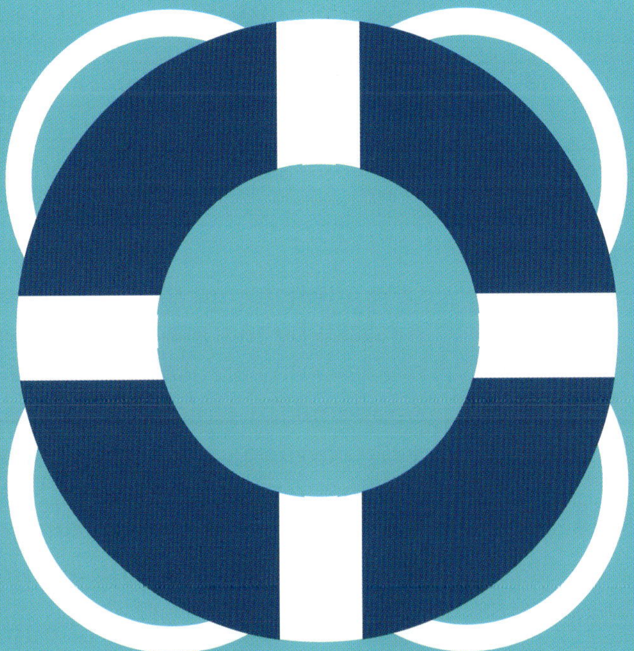

11 While there is no consistent definition of a small vessel, most jurisdictions consider small vessels to be those from 5–8 metres in length.

There are few rigorous studies to guide many of the activities in this section, though there is clear evidence that compulsory, government-approved lifejacket-wearing regulations (applicable to small boats rather than large ships or ferries) are successful in reducing drowning deaths *(81–84)*. The lack of rigorous study underlines the importance of ensuring that evaluation accompanies any new boating, shipping or ferry safety measure in order to add to the evidence base. This section separately addresses the needs of large and small vessels.

Large vessels

Between 2000 and 2014 approximately 23 000 lives were lost in ferry accidents worldwide. Ninety-four percent of these deaths occurred in developing countries, with almost 9000 ferry -related fatalities in South and South-East Asia, and 6000 in East and West Africa *(85)*.

Setting and enforcing safe shipping and ferry regulations

⇩ Step one

Assess the situation

See page 5

An assessment (see Situational assessment) may include: the number of at-risk persons and vessels; the number of drowning events; and all recorded safety risk management issues (for example, lifejackets that are not accessible or used for another purpose on the boat). Remember that responsibility for shipping legislation, licensing and enforcement may be shared by several ministries.

⇩ Step two

Train operators to competent and professional standards

One study found that human error – defined broadly as any mistake by mariners (or passengers) that causes or exacerbates an accident – was linked to 85% of all large ferry accidents for which a cause could be determined (for example overcrowding, poor route planning or poor cargo stowage leading to vessel instability) *(85)*. Governments can combat this by improving operator and crew training and certification processes, and properly enforcing robust safety regulations.

To minimize the impact of human error on ferries in particular, ferry owners and operators must establish a safety culture – a top-down, bottom-up commitment to safety similar to that created by the airline industry, where safety is everyone's business (and passengers are shown how to use a lifejacket on each journey), and learning from accidents is prioritized.

Ferry owners and operators must establish a safety culture – a top-down, bottom-up commitment to safety similar to that created by the airline industry, where safety is everyone's business.

Training is one way to do this. Training on safety management systems helps crews manage risks, including human and mechanical factors, tides, currents and weather conditions. E-learning (use of electronic devices for self-study) that supplements, or potentially replaces, expensive off-site training and self-funded study is a cost-effective, efficient way to help mariners learn and get feedback on their proficiency. E-learning is most effective when blended with on-board training. The Bangladesh Department of Shipping, Interferry and the International Maritime Organization (IMO) successfully trialled (without further continuation) a CD-based course in 2006. Building on this experience, the Worldwide Ferry Safety Association is planning an e-learning course using mobile devices, working with several partners in developing countries.

⇩ Step three

Improve detection and dissemination of information about the weather

Bad weather has played a role in more than 50% of all fatal ferry accidents worldwide since 2000 *(85)*. Reducing fatalities associated with bad weather can benefit from new, innovative and affordable weather forecasting, monitoring and dissemination techniques, and these can be adopted by state and private operators.

Weather detection and dissemination techniques have improved markedly in high-income countries, many of which can be accessed by low- and middle-income countries. Technologies such as 3D printed weather monitors – the first five of which have been set up in Zambia *(86)* – assist weather detection in remote locations *(87)*,[12] while the USA's National Oceanic and Atmospheric Administration's GOES-R satellite is set to provide frequent, high-resolution updates of weather conditions and track hazardous weather conditions in the western hemisphere. Countries in the regions it covers will be able to sign up to weather alerts when the satellite is launched (due in 2016). This will set the standard for subsequent high-quality weather monitoring satellites *(88)*. SMS-based weather alert systems have been established and used in Bangladesh to disseminate crucial weather information *(89, 90)*.

12 This technology has been developed by the University of Cooperative Atmospheric Research, funded by the USA's National Oceanic and Atmospheric Administration (NOAA) programme.

⇩ Step four

Adopt technologies and incentives that promote adherence to regulations for proper loading of vessels

Overcrowding contributed to around 30% of all ferry fatality accidents between 2000–2014 *(85)*. In some cases vessels were two or three times over the safe passenger limit. Incomplete passenger manifests (sometimes used to conceal overcrowding) made accurate fatality counts impossible for some accidents. Correct passenger counting, either manually (for low- and middle-income countries) or with crowd-counting technology can prevent overcrowding, potentially reducing accidents.

All ferry operators:

- should put in place passenger and vehicle-counting measures commensurate with vessel size and manufacturers' recommendations;
- could use mobile phone ticketing (where passengers obtain tickets via a mobile phone or handset) to ensure that there are enough vessels to accommodate all passengers to whom tickets have been sold.

Governments and local authorities should:

- consider subsidies for ferry operators in developing countries who find it difficult to remain financially viable (a situation exacerbated by non-economic government tariffs placed on them), thereby reducing the incentive for overcrowding;
- conduct spot checks to ensure compliance with vessel manufacturers' and operators' guidelines.

⇩ Step five

Ensure vessels are fit for purpose

Many passenger vessels – whether second-hand, locally constructed or repurposed from other countries or sectors – are not inspected by regulatory bodies and may be poorly maintained.

Governments must:

- implement basic inspection and approval processes to ensure vessels conform as appropriate to the IMO's regulatory framework and conventions *(91)*, and enforce robust safety regulations;
- ensure compliance with such processes as a pre-condition of financial or other development assistance, particularly where such assistance is given to the maritime transport sector;

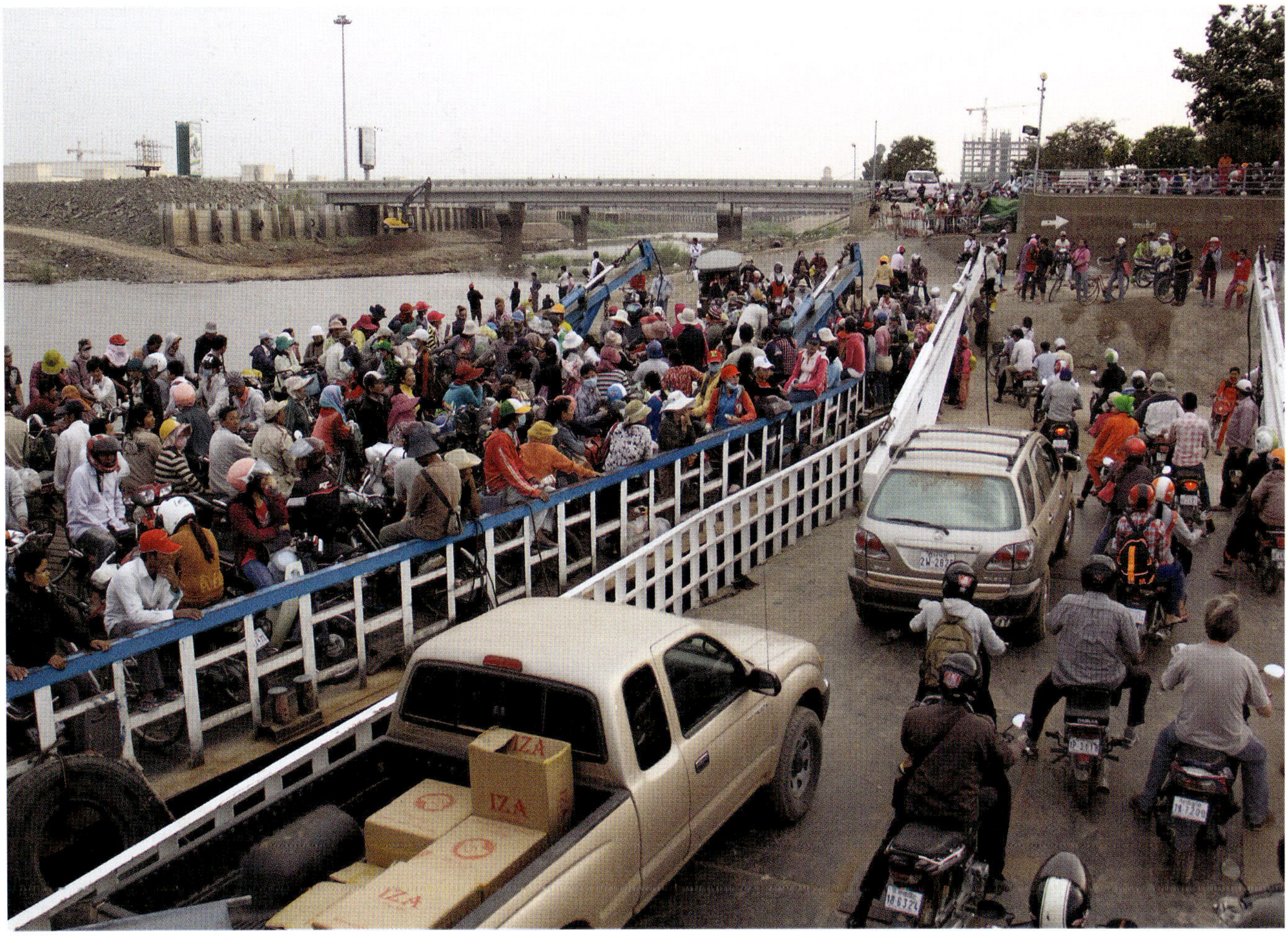

Overcrowding contributed to around 30% of all ferry fatality accidents between 2000–2014.

- educate operators on routine maintenance and train them to perform pre-trip checks and vessel maintenance tasks;
- ensure safety officers or water police perform vessel safety spot checks at launch sites.

International and national authorities and professional associations should:

- encourage the design and manufacture of safe, affordable, waterway-appropriate ferries;
- ensure adequate lifejackets and life rafts for all passengers and crew, with well-rehearsed safety plans to ensure the crew can manage the call to "abandon ship";
- ensure effective (and serviced) fire-fighting appliances, and crews trained in their use.

Small vessels

The number of deaths related to small vessels worldwide is unknown as very few data are collected on boating-related drowning, which mainly occurs during occupational fishing and water transport in low- and middle-income countries.

Governments can combat human error as a cause of drowning by improving operator and crew training and certification processes, and properly enforcing robust safety regulations.

One review of a small-scale vessel registration system for Pacific island countries and territories conducted in 2016 revealed that passengers on small vessels used for fishing or inter-island transport are at increased risk of drowning due to vessel instability, potential lack of safety and communications equipment, and extreme weather events. The review found that while seven of 14 Pacific island countries and territories had enacted some form of small-vessel registration scheme, poor agency coordination, resourcing and training, inconsistencies in small vessel definition and financial deterrents all affected the success of registration as a safety strategy in the region *(92)*.

Major modifiable risk factors for all boating deaths in high-income countries are non-use of lifejackets, use of alcohol by boat operators and passengers, and lack of on-board safety equipment *(93, 94)*. Some high-income countries have established national or state recreational boating incident and injury data collection systems, and each year report the number of boating-related deaths and contributing factors.

Setting and enforcing safe boating regulations

Step one

Assess the situation

See page 5

As part of your situational assessment (see Situational assessment), remember that responsibility for boating legislation, licensing and regulation enforcement may be the responsibility of more than one ministry, or the sector may be entirely unregulated or unsupervised.

Step two

Train operators to competent and professional standards

Aspects of human error were among the top five contributing factors to recreational boating accidents in the USA in 2014 *(95)*. Governments can combat human error as a cause of drowning by improving operator and crew training and certification processes, and properly enforcing robust safety regulations. Training is one element of improving safety (see examples in Box 7), and helps fisherfolk and other small-boat operators to manage risks, including human and mechanical factors, tides, currents and weather conditions. Measures include:

- education – vessel operator licensing schemes (knowledge and practical tests including retrieval of man overboard);
- regulation – safe vessel operation regulations, including mandatory carrying of safety equipment appropriate for vessel and waterway type – e.g. torch, bailer, bucket and lanyard, lifebuoy, distress beacon, flares, marine radio etc.;
- enforcement – spot checks of operator licences.

Step three

Limit alcohol and illicit drug use among small boat operators

Reducing or eliminating alcohol and illicit drug use by boaters addresses a key drowning risk factor. This can be done through:

See page 75

- public awareness campaigns around drowning risk and prevention, and boater/small boat operator education about existing regulations (see Strengthen public awareness);
- regulations that limit or ban alcohol and drug use in watersports and fishing environments;
- enforcement of laws through random breath checks on the water at launch sites and policing local regulations banning public alcohol use in watersports and fishing environments *(96)*.

Box 7: Training schemes in Australia, Canada, USA

Many jurisdictions in high-income countries such as Australia, Canada and the USA have introduced recreational boat operator licensing schemes. This is an attempt to improve vessel operators' basic knowledge and understanding of the rules and the safety requirements of operating small, motorized boats, and what to do in an emergency. In most of these jurisdictions, boaters are required to pass a boating safety knowledge test that is usually taken at the end of a training course delivered by accredited course providers. Some jurisdictions offer online courses.

The state of Western Australia is one of the few jurisdictions to include a requirement that boat operators pass a practical test – boaters are required to show competency in a set series of practical skills when operating a vessel over a 1-hour boating trip. There are no published evaluations on the effectiveness of licensing schemes, and where they do exist they rely on the pre-existence of at least some level of regulatory framework and enforcement.

⇩ Step four

Promote regulations for proper loading of vessels

A recent study in Uganda revealed improper loading and/or overloading was one of three most frequently mentioned factors linked to capsizing and drowning *(97)*. Measures to reduce the risk of improper loading or overloading include:

- educating operators on safe vessel loading and stability;
- establishing rules on safe loading and maximum carrying capacity of vessels (based on vessel length/manufacturers' recommendations);
- spot checks of compliance with manufacturers' and operators' guidelines.

⇩ Step five

Ensure vessels are fit for purpose

Recent studies estimate that wearing a lifejacket may at least halve recreational boating drowning deaths in high-income countries.

Governments must develop and enforce safety standards for the manufacture of small vessels (including measures to improve buoyancy and stability) and promote regular vessel maintenance and pre-trip checks by the operator. Measures include:

- educating operators on routine maintenance, training them to perform pre-trip checks and vessel maintenance tasks;
- developing and enforcing safety standards for the manufacture of small vessels that include measures to improve buoyancy and stability;
- vessel safety checks at launch sites.

⇩ Step six

Improve detection and dissemination of information about the weather

A key measure to prevent drowning is to reduce vessel operation in hazardous weather conditions and equip vessels to respond to sudden adverse weather conditions. Measures include:

- developing weather alert systems to inform vessel operators of local weather forecasts and sudden changes in conditions;
- increasing boat operator and passenger access to weather reports and alerts.

⇩ Step seven

Regulate and enforce mandatory wearing of lifejackets in high-income countries and encourage and support expansion of their use in low- and middle-income counties

Recent studies estimate that wearing a lifejacket may at least halve recreational boating drowning deaths in high-income countries *(98, 99)* (similar studies have not been conducted in low- and middle-income countries). Educational campaigns promoting lifejacket use have produced limited and short-term effects but mandatory lifejacket-wearing regulations combined with boater education and enforcement have resulted in large and sustained increases in lifejacket wearing among both child and adult boaters on small boats *(100, 101)*.

When designing interventions to increase lifejacket wearing, barriers to their use and to community and boater acceptance of mandatory regulations should be researched and addressed. For example, the cost of approved lifejackets is a major barrier in low-resource communities living close to water in high-income countries, and to fisherfolk and the general population using small boats for transport in low- and middle-income countries *(97)*. Solutions include subsidized lifejackets, lifejacket loan schemes and free lifejacket distribution programmes. Design and technology innovations can also increase comfort, ease of use and acceptance of lifejackets *(102, 103)*. Low-cost, locally made designs have also been trialled in some communities.

See page 30

Socio-cultural factors in high-income countries contributing to poor or inconsistent lifejacket use among boaters include low perception of drowning risk (especially in calm conditions), the perception that lifejackets are uncomfortable and unattractive *(104)* and the belief that wearing a lifejacket indicates user inexperience or poor swimming ability *(104)*. These factors can be addressed through education (see Teach school-aged children swimming and water safety).

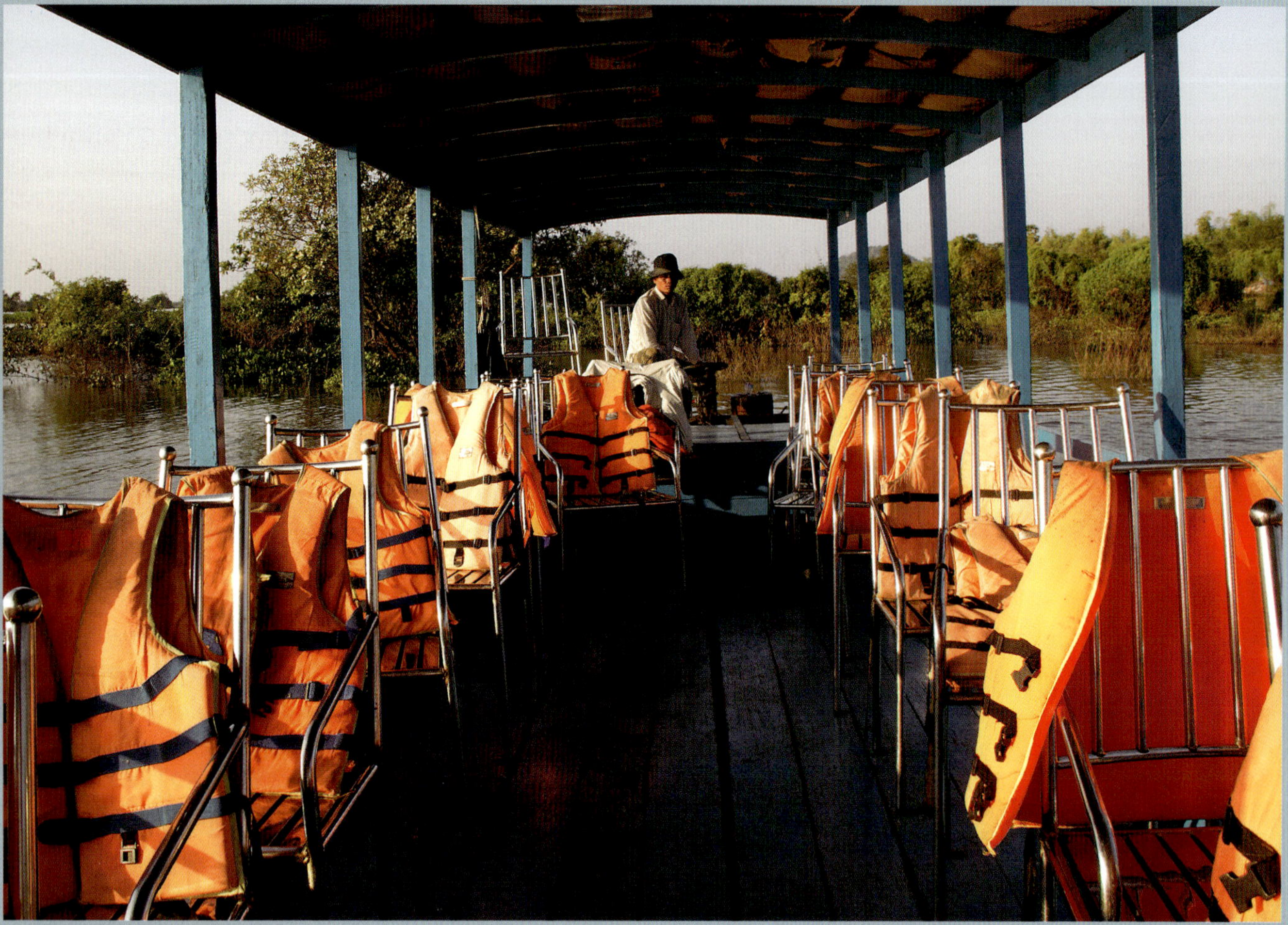

Case study

Mandatory lifejacket regulations reduce drowning deaths, Victoria, Australia

Comprehensive and mandatory lifejacket-wearing regulations adopted in Victoria, Australia, in 2005 significantly decreased boater drowning deaths *(98)*, with 59 recreational boating drowning deaths in the 6-year pre-intervention period (1998 to 2004) compared to 16 in the 5-year post-intervention period (2005 to 2010).

The major trigger for the regulations was the State Coroner's public recommendation in 2003 that the marine regulator, Marine Safety Victoria (MSV), mandate lifejacket wearing for all occupants of recreational vessels at all times. This was prompted by a coronial study of regional boater drowning deaths mainly involving vessels under 6 metres in length, where lifejackets were either not available or unable to be used because of sudden immersion *(85)*.

MSV entered a 2-year period of education and consultation with key industry groups, boating and water sports organizations, boaters and the public to negotiate the parameters of lifejacket regulations. The proposed regulations were refined (for example the proposed vessel length cut-off for compulsory wear was reduced from 6 metres to 4.8 metres) to meet informed criticism and build political, stakeholder and community support.

Search and rescue related to vessels of all sizes

Improved search and rescue (SAR) capability reduces fatalities associated with large and small vessels alike. The International Maritime Rescue Federation (IMRF) seeks to improve SAR capability worldwide, and in particular the provision of:

- adequate training and equipment, including reliable emergency alerting devices and basic survival equipment;
- adequate communications facilities, so that emergency alerts can be received and SAR facilities tasked and coordinated;
- adequate SAR capability for "normal" emergencies – lacking in many parts of the world;
- mass-rescue operations capability which, as defined by the IMO, requires special planning by relevant authorities.

Improved search and rescue (SAR) capability reduces fatalities associated with large and small vessels alike.

IMRF provides resources to help address these concerns (see www.international-maritime-rescue.org for more information), and the *International Aeronautical and Maritime Search and Rescue (IAMSAR) Manual*, published by the IMO and the International Civil Aviation Organization, is also a useful resource.

Measures to achieve improved SAR capability include the following:

- **Planning and resourcing (locally and nationally)** should include identifying the SAR resources available, including coordination and communications systems, and, based on sound risk assessment, should identify what additional resources are required to find and rescue people in distress.
- **Public awareness and action** to identify at-risk groups locally and develop effective educational, regulatory and safety and emergency equipment provision strategies.
- **Multisectoral collaboration** is essential in maritime emergency response, especially in mass-rescue operations: a national SAR committee is recommended (see the IAMSAR manual).
- **Monitoring and evaluation/research** is required to illuminate currently under-explored areas such as quantifying the number of lives lost at sea each year; identifying higher-risk areas, geographically and by activity sector; and analysing the effectiveness of response strategies.

Section 3

Strategies to support drowning prevention interventions

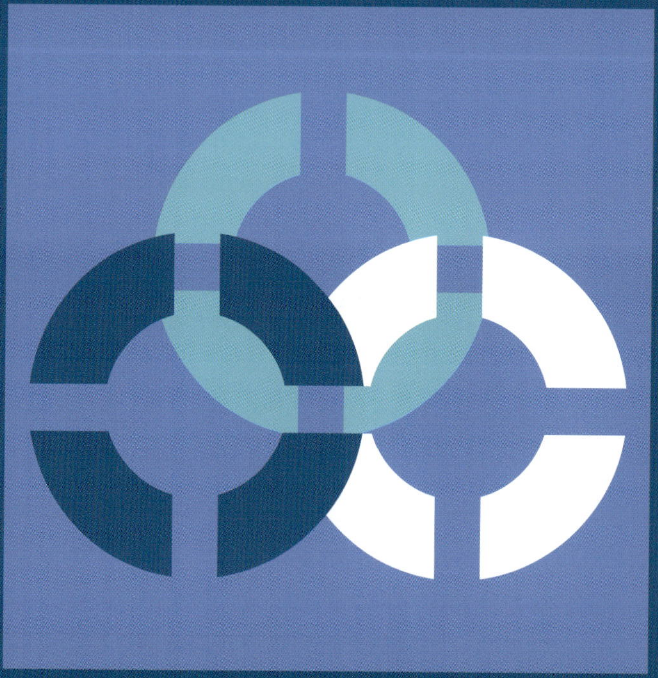

1
Promote multisectoral collaboration
Page 67

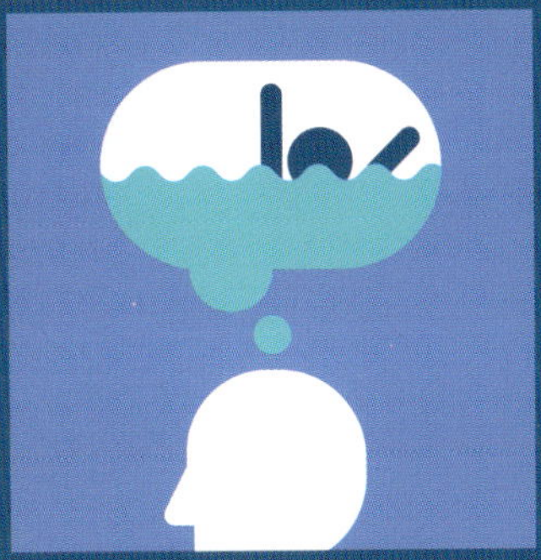

2

Strengthen public awareness of drowning through strategic communications

Page 75

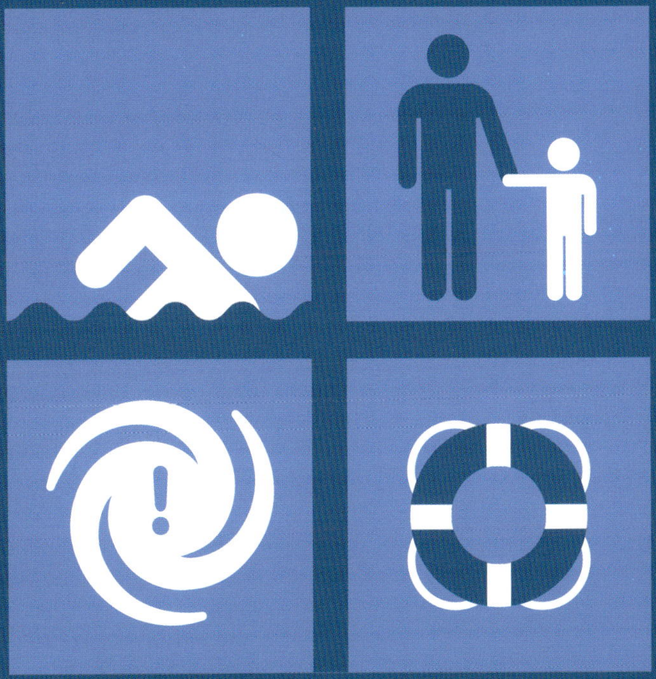

3

Establish a national water safety (drowning prevention) plan

Page 81

4

Research: advance drowning prevention through data collection and well-designed studies

Page 89

1
Promote multisectoral collaboration

Multisectoral collaboration means working with other interested parties to achieve a goal. While not all parties may have drowning prevention as their primary goal, their agendas and activities may nevertheless intersect and help reduce drowning deaths. Including drowning prevention interventions may also help other parties achieve their goals.

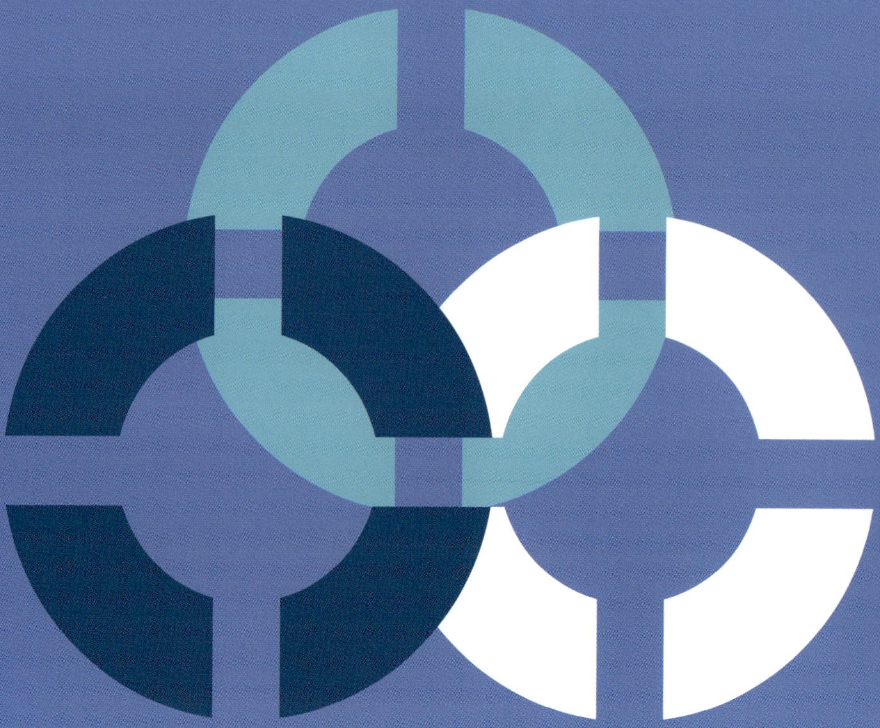

Benefits of multisectoral collaboration

Most countries lack the infrastructure to coordinate drowning prevention efforts. This contrasts, for example, with road safety, for which (in some countries) dedicated ministries and government departments have a stated responsibility. The lack of such an over-arching, responsible body partly explains the limited action to date on drowning prevention in many countries, but also suggests that multisectoral collaboration is a proven strategy for progress.

See page 81

Multisectoral collaboration can align or integrate aspects of drowning prevention with various sectors' current jurisdictional responsibilities and objectives without diminishing its importance. At national level, a "whole-of-government" approach can encompass all necessary sectors in a coordinated strategy and action plan (see Establish a national water safety plan), and monitor progress and accountability of the implementation process. Similar collaborations may need to be replicated at local or regional level to achieve coordinated effort and to bring successful local interventions to scale following evaluation.

Who needs to be involved?

See page 74

Multisectoral collaboration involving government, NGOs, the health-care sector, researchers, the media, industry and civil society groups is vital for effective drowning prevention at local, regional and national level. A matrix can be used to set out the roles of sectors in relation to the various drowning issues (see Table 3). Such a matrix could be drawn up for activities at all levels, with clear indicators of what the collaboration aims to achieve.

Opportunities for multisectoral collaboration

Multisectoral collaboration on drowning prevention happens where different sectors' agendas intersect – for example:

- on specific drowning-related issues such as maritime safety, managing flood risks, day care in low-resource settings or safe-water and sanitation provision;
- following the introduction of international frameworks, for example the Sustainable Development Goals (SDGs), or during the development of whole-of-government national water safety strategies or plans;
- during disaster responses (floods, tsunamis, major maritime disasters), or following high-profile drowning deaths;
- on publication of formal reports by health, shipping, safety, and national security inspectorates etc.

See page 74

Issue-oriented collaborations

While government sectors can potentially coordinate, support, finance and monitor drowning prevention efforts, specific issue-oriented collaborations will benefit all interventions in this guide (i.e. vessels, day care, swim skills, rescue and resuscitation, barriers and floods), and will include many nongovernmental actors (see Table 3). Collaboration on drowning prevention for large and small vessels would require a different set of collaborators, for example, to those needed to develop swimming programmes or flood control and early warning systems.

Another good intersectoral example is the major water, sanitation and health agenda to increase the number of people worldwide who have drinking water from sources protected from outside contamination. People using them are less likely to drown in them than they are if using surface water or open wells. Similarly, controlling water-borne diseases by draining or filling in unwanted ditches, waterholes or ponds also reduces exposure to drowning risks.

Controlling water-borne diseases by draining or filling in unwanted ditches, waterholes or ponds... reduces exposure to drowning risks.

International framework collaborations

SDG 9, to "build resilient infrastructure, promote sustainable industrialization and foster innovation", and SDG 6, Target 6.1, "by 2030, achieve universal and equitable access to safe and affordable drinking water for all" aim to provide contamination-free drinking water; this offers good opportunities for multisectoral collaboration around drowning prevention because a safe, local supply of drinking water not only improves health and sanitation, but also eliminates the collection of water from high drowning risk locations such as rivers, streams and uncovered wells. Similarly, tap water delivered directly to homes eliminates the need for storage in buckets and large vessels – common locations for infant and toddler drowning. Additionally, building resilient infrastructure may provide flood protection.

Disasters and time-dependent responses

Rapid, often national and international responses from multiple sectors are required for rescue and harm-minimization following water disasters such as floods and tsunamis. Water-related disasters are nearly instantly fatal when they strike. Embedding early warning, awareness, self-rescue and rescue of others skills within the at-risk community prior to the event is probably the best way to reduce drowning mortality. Secondary prevention strategies are less effective and more challenging.

Another area for collaboration is meeting media requests for information following a drowning. Timely provision of relevant drowning data is an opportunity to get evidence-based information on drowning prevention included in media coverage following a drowning event.

Implementing multisectoral collaboration for drowning prevention

Establishing multisectoral collaborations and conducting a needs assessment for drowning interventions require an integrated process and benefit from broad, inclusive, sectoral and key-player recruitment and engagement. The following steps are suggested as a guide.

Step one

Identify and connect with stakeholders

See pages 74 and 5

Often drowning prevention is absent from the government agenda. Consider creating a matrix of potential collaborators that have jurisdictional or organizational ownership of the problem and/or solutions, and identify common ground, shared agendas or interests, and potential benefits to sectors and collaborators (see Table 3 and Situational assessment). Connect with potential participating organizations, government officials, individuals and civil society networks and invite them to collaborate. Request that all participants bring the appropriate level of decision-making responsibility, collaborative behaviour and knowledge to the partnership.

Step two

Identify or create opportunities for collaboration

Identify, create or anticipate windows of opportunity for collaboration. Prepare implementation plans for evidence-based drowning prevention interventions so opportunities can be seized when these coincide with policy agendas, or when public recognition of the problem of drowning is heightened (for instance when drowning tragedies happen or when data on high drowning rates are published).

Step three

Identify your chosen framework, goals, leadership and roles

Make sure your framework aligns with existing policies, frameworks and infrastructure that address your chosen issue or potential solutions. Identify an appropriate political or government leader or other high profile "champion" of drowning prevention to host an initial meeting and to invite selected or nominated attendees. Decide which agencies would lead and be accountable for components of the intervention.

⇩ Step four

Establish sustainability

Integrate drowning prevention into relevant sectors' policies, job descriptions, key performance indicators and ongoing funding streams.

⇩ Step five

Establish terms of reference

Identify broad approaches to reach your goals and potentially set targets for a reduction in the drowning rate (including proven intermediate measures such as lifejacket wearing in small boats; or proportion of primary school children who have received swim skills and water safety training).

⇩ Step six

Ensure appropriate resources

See page 5

See page 89

Engage stakeholders with the resources and influence to maximize the impact of drowning prevention work, such as relevant government departments, high-profile swimming champions, the media and relevant industries, and ensure the work is appropriately supported by government and other partners such as NGOs. This will more likely be achieved where the size of the problem and the social and economic cost can be described (see Situational assessment), alongside evidence-based solutions (see Research).

⇩ Step seven

Create an environment for scaling-up successful interventions

See page 89

See page 75

Ensuring that interventions are rigorously evaluated and results published in peer-reviewed literature wherever possible (see Research) is a key strategy to promote the scaling-up of drowning prevention interventions. Apart from peer-reviewed studies, reports to government and the media, bringing aboard "champions" for the cause, and strong advocacy (including behaviour-change campaigns run across various media, see Strengthen public awareness) can all be used to bring effective interventions to scale. Strategic aspects to focus on in order to get drowning prevention on the government's agenda include evidence of cost-effectiveness (drawing on data that illustrate the drowning burden), sustainability of interventions, and pathways for bringing to scale (see case study, page 76).

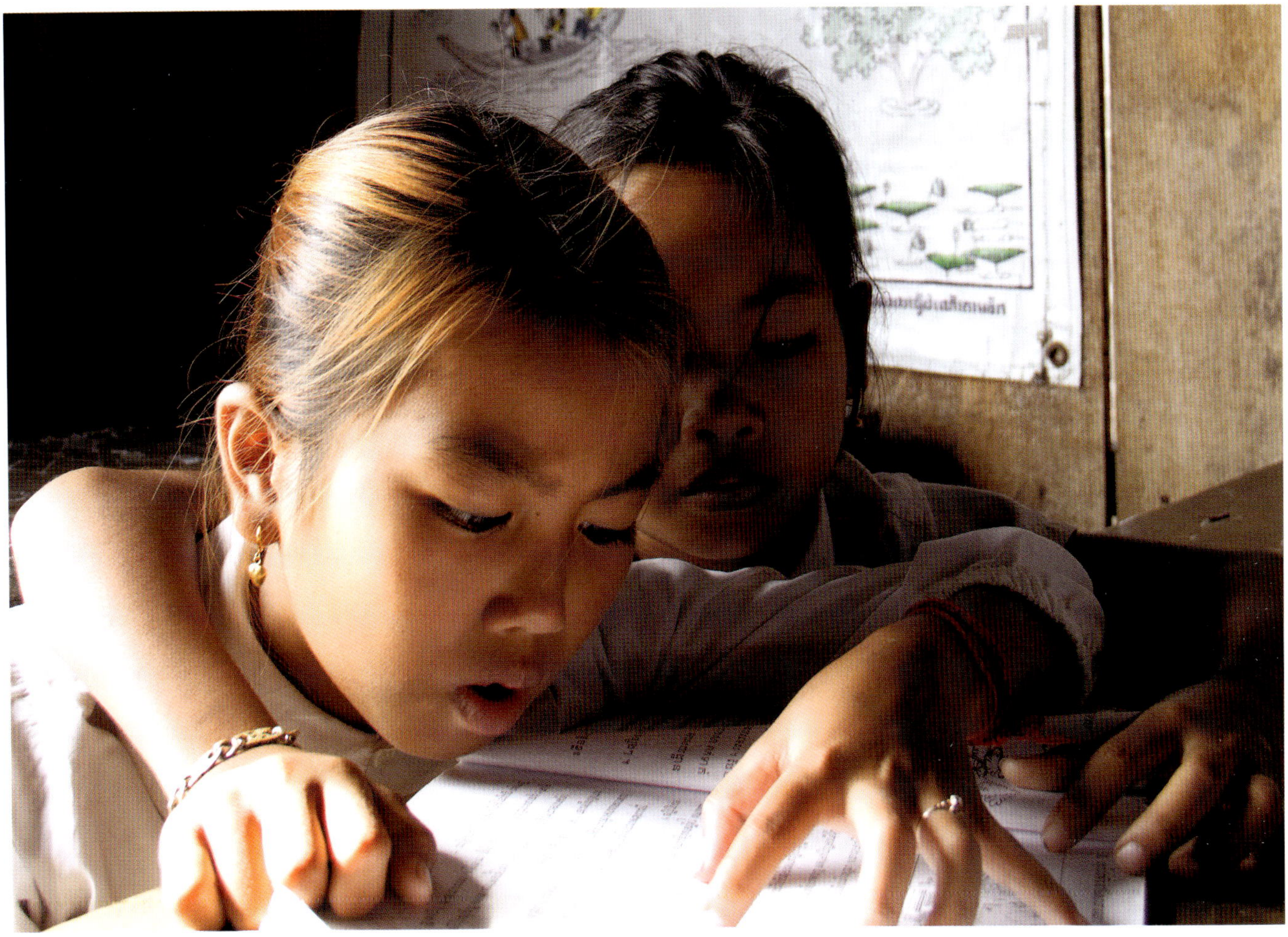

⇩ Step eight

Contribute to international policy development

See page 75

Collaborations should discuss and develop powerful and cohesive messaging (see Strengthen public awareness), and use this to inform international agencies and donors about the size and social and economic costs of drowning. Efforts of larger collaborations and partnerships should seek inclusion of drowning prevention on the agendas of United Nations agencies, international NGOs and donor agencies. To be effective it may first be necessary to make the case at national level (drawing on data on countries' drowning burden) so that drowning is also represented among countries' priorities in discussions with international agencies.

⇩ Step nine

Monitor and evaluate

Review the effectiveness of the collaboration against its terms of reference and decide which agency (typically a university), study design and baseline data are required to evaluate the intervention.

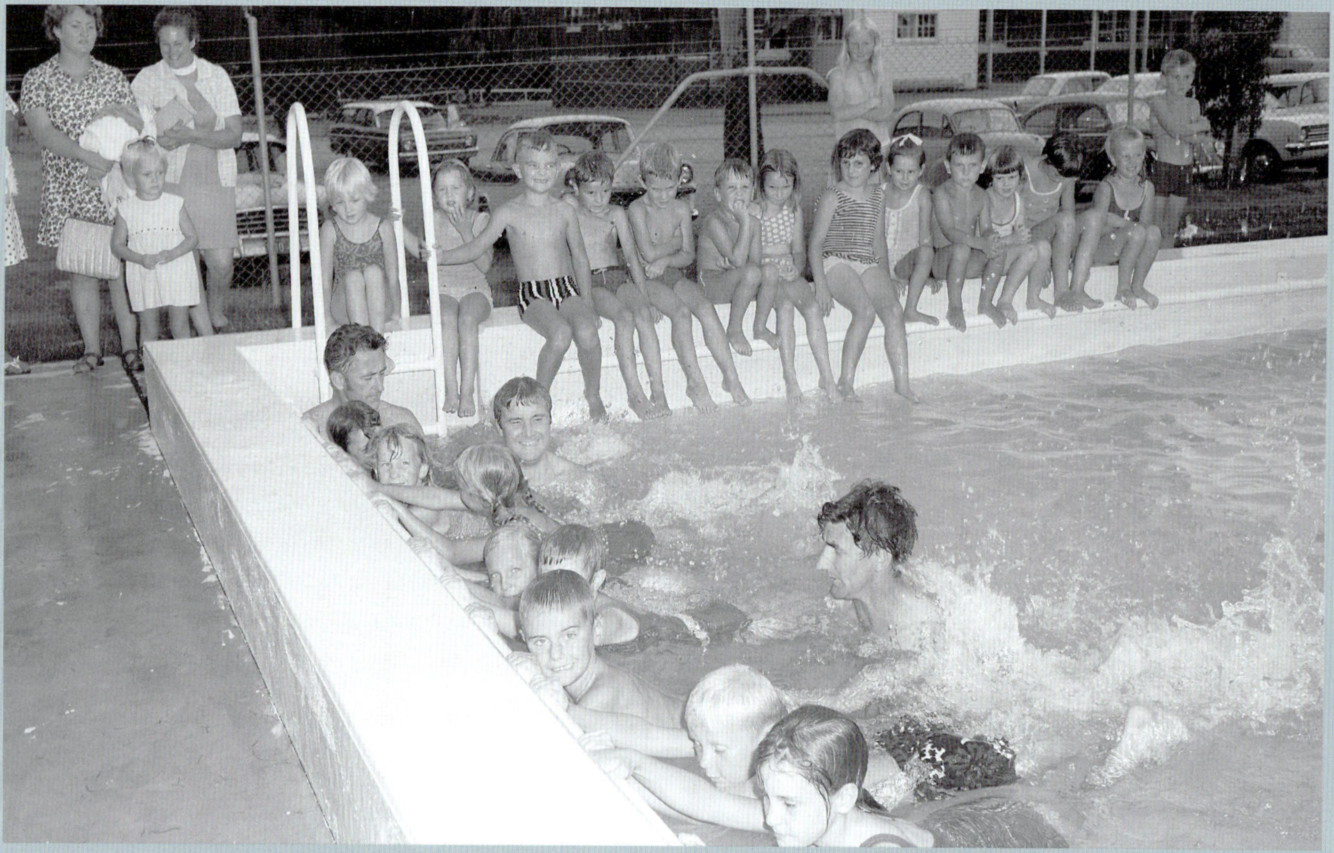

Case study

Successful (free) swim programme scaled-up to the whole-child population, Australia

In 1906, in the state of Victoria, Australia, the newly established Royal Life Saving Society responded to persistently high drowning rates by calling for swimming lessons for children. Fledgling swim clubs and learn-to-swim programmes emerged, and the Education Department systematically contributed to progress by 1910. Two important "champions" drove progress over several decades – a dedicated teacher who taught other teachers to swim and who, in turn, taught children to swim (a process that peaked with 5000 certified swim-trainer teachers by the mid-1950s), and a high-profile Olympic swimmer. The *Herald* newspaper added support and publicity in 1928, and, despite many barriers, swimming programmes had increased moderately by the middle of the century.

The 1956 Melbourne Olympic Games provided new impetus. Local governments, the Education Department, lifesaving societies, volunteers and the *Herald* newspaper collaborated in the *Herald* Learn to Swim campaign, teaching more than 80 000 children to swim each year by 1961 (and a total of 1 million by 1963). The collaborative effect of swim teaching, building community pools and increased public awareness was associated with significant drowning reductions. While there may have been other contributing factors, during the intervening 60 years the drowning rate in Victoria for children aged 5–14 years fell from 18.7 per 100 000 to 3.7 per 100 000 for boys and 2.6 per 100 000 to 1.7 per 100 000 for girls.

Today, because of the early stages of development of drowning prevention globally, there are few examples of successful scaling-up of effective interventions, particularly those that involve behavioural and organizational change. This case study demonstrates many of the key points about multisectoral collaboration at play. It also demonstrates that, like many public health advances, full scale-up took several decades. It is possible that such progress could be accelerated, with current knowledge, in low- and middle-income countries, where drowning rates remain high *(105)*.

Table 3: Sample matrix of potential national collaborators and contributions

Sector	Marine/small boats	Swimming	Rescue and resuscitation	Barriers and hazard removal	Floods and development	Cross-sectoral and general
Government	Implementation of best practice legislation, regulations and enforcement for large and small vessel safety Refugee safety Safe water-transport to school and work	Providing safe places to swim Swimming and water safety programmes	Rescue and resuscitation programmes	Child safety in the home Safe drinking water programmes	Implement SDG 9: Build resilient infrastructure	Implement relevant *Global report on drowning* actions; relevant SDGs Collect and make available all relevant drowning data Develop a national drowning prevention strategy Finance drowning prevention Community awareness and education programmes
NGOs	Advocacy and technical expertise (e.g. lifejackets) Safe water transport to school and work	Nationally accredited swimming and water safety programmes	Rescue and resuscitation programmes	Child safety in the home Safe drinking water programmes	Advocacy; provision of safe drinking water (and drowning prevention) programmes	Implement relevant recommendations from the WHO *Global report on drowning* Contribute to national strategy
Media	Dissemination of information, advocacy	Dissemination of information	Dissemination of information	Dissemination of information	Warnings Dissemination of information	Contribute to national strategy Journalist training on issues and advocacy role for prevention
Industry, private sector	Safe innovative boat design. Safe and effective lifejacket design	Nationally accredited swim skill and water safety programmes; training swim teachers; lifeguards	Rescue and resuscitation development and training	Community education programmes		Contribute to national strategy
Tertiary education sector						Apply drowning data quality standards; analyse data; conduct research and evaluation studies Inclusion of drowning prevention in tertiary education courses such as engineering, agricultural science, public health and education

2

Strengthen public awareness of drowning through strategic communications

Public awareness and behaviour change campaigns are crucial if drowning prevention measures are to be accepted and successful. Indeed, in many settings people are not even aware that drowning is a major problem. Therefore, strategic communications should be integrated into the planning phase of all interventions.

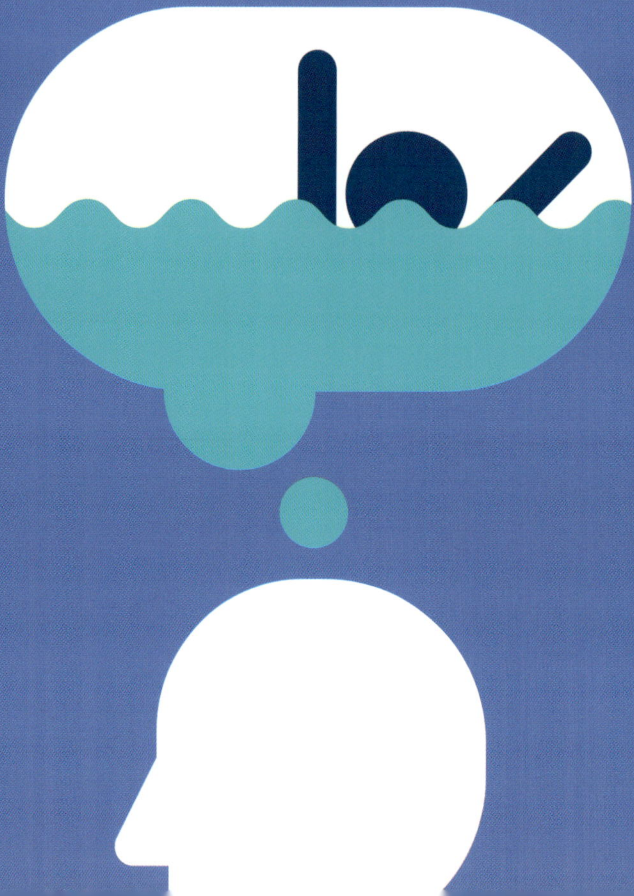

Benefits of strategic communications in raising awareness of drowning

Strategic communications include **public awareness** campaigns targeting the general population and decision-makers, and **behaviour change campaigns** aimed at specific communities or risk groups. These strategies help drowning prevention efforts engage a wide range of stakeholders and achieve their goals, by, among others: promoting new policies; enforcing regulations; implementing concrete physical measures; and ensuring communities' acceptance and use of new drowning prevention resources (particularly those that protect children).

Strengthening public awareness using strategic communications

Effective strategic communications depend on understanding what people believe and why they behave as they do.

The six drowning prevention interventions set out in this guide are varied but have similarities: all are implemented by stakeholders at different levels (national and local) and all require behaviour change communications at community level. Many will require public awareness campaigns among the general population. All campaigns – whether for awareness raising or behavioural change – should include these steps *(106)*.

⇩ Step one

Assess the potential for strategic communications

Effective strategic communications depend on understanding **what** people believe and **why** they behave as they do, based on factors such as their existing knowledge and perceptions, the local environment, social norms, a perception of the risk, and beliefs about their power (or lack of power) to change things. Behaviours are also the product of how people evaluate their choices in terms of costs, benefits and barriers – whether these barriers are perceived or actual, internal or external, tangible or intangible, monetary or non-monetary *(107)*.

It is critical to assess this as a first step, using tools such as focus group discussions and knowledge, attitudes and practices (KAP) surveys. Example questions to answer using these tools include: what do people know and believe about drowning? Who do parents trust, and can those people share information about drowning? Why is day care accepted in some communities but not others? What type of information is needed, when, where and why? Action that the community has taken in the past can often provide a starting point.

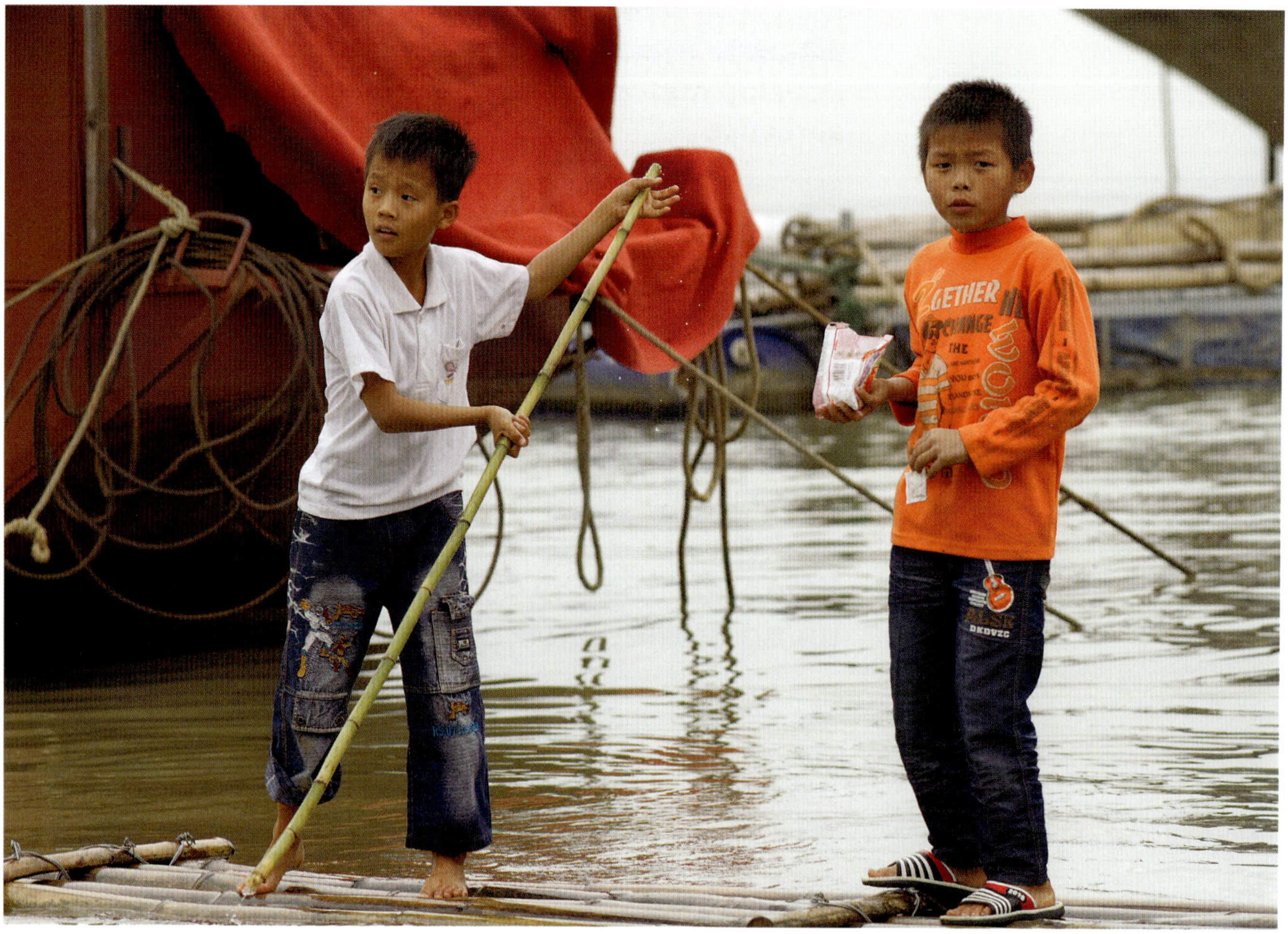

Messages should be based on insight gathered in the research phase and refer to target audiences' existing knowledge and beliefs.

⇩ Step two

Define audience

Defining the target audience and narrowing the focus to a particular at risk group (such as parents of young children or population groups with higher rates of drowning) is key for an effective communications strategy.

⇩ Step three

Define the strategy

The situational assessment in step 1 will inform the selection of messages, media and channels. Several methods exist to create to behaviour-change messages: for example, messages can be focused on presenting the benefit of the desired behaviour or the negative consequences of the problem behaviour. Behaviour-change campaigns should coordinate with enforcement where relevant, for example on small vessel regulations, pool fencing, etc.

Step four

Develop materials and messages relevant to the target audience

Messages should be based on insight gathered in the research phase and refer to target audiences' existing knowledge and beliefs. Likewise, the selection of materials used to disseminate the messages should reflect the target audience's preference and habits. A campaign may have different target audiences and stakeholders, and therefore require different messages and communication platforms. Messages and materials should be tested through focus groups before being disseminated.

Step five

Disseminate materials and messages

Depending on the campaign's objectives and target audience, messages can be disseminated through a variety of channels, such as traditional media (print, billboards, television, radio); culturally specific media (community theatre, puppetry, debates, song and dance, riddles, proverbs); "edutainment"; social and digital media; public events; community mobilization; activities in schools and colleges; engagement of community leaders or other key groups; promotion of free or subsidized goods such as lifejackets for boaters; news articles on mass media, etc. A variety of channels is better than one main channel.

Step six

Evaluate the campaign

See page 89

Communications efforts can be evaluated at different levels. For example, post-campaign surveys evaluate a campaign's reach and recall, and concretely define how many people have seen or heard the campaign and took away the key message. Evaluations can also be done to define the impact of the campaign and the intervention on behaviour (see Research). For this type of evaluation it is important to conduct a pre-campaign baseline survey that can be compared with the post-campaign survey evaluation.

The following sample campaign to equip ferries with lifejackets illustrates how strategic communications may be used to catalyze the need for, and later support implementation of, the intervention:

- **Phase 1:** The campaign selects legislators and regulators as the audience to target for a change in laws and policies related to lifejackets on ferries. As part of this awareness raising and advocacy campaign, messages on the magnitude of the problem (evidenced through a pre-campaign survey of current practice) and the benefit of the intervention – equipping ferries with quality lifejackets – are shared though mass media articles (traditional and digital) and targeted at technical meetings with stakeholders.

- **Phase 2 (post legislation):** The campaign targets a second audience, ferry operators, to increase compliance with new legislation on lifejackets on ferries. Messages focus on strict enforcement of the new law or on possible benefits for the company if consumers associate it with safety. These messages are disseminated through articles in ferry industry publications; presentations at companies' boards of directors; meetings with ferry companies' marketing teams; and posters and print publications disseminated at the companies' premises.
- **Phase 3:** The campaign targets its third audience, ferry users, to increase demand for on-board safety. Messages focus on consumers' right to safe travel, the importance of checking safety features before purchasing services from one provider or another, the magnitude of the problem and the effectiveness of quality lifejackets. Messages are disseminated through mass media (television, radio or print material), articles on news media, brochures, posters and fliers available at ticket centres (and on ferries), as well as through awareness raising groups engaging with travellers in ports. Travellers at ports can be engaged to complete a post-campaign survey of practice.

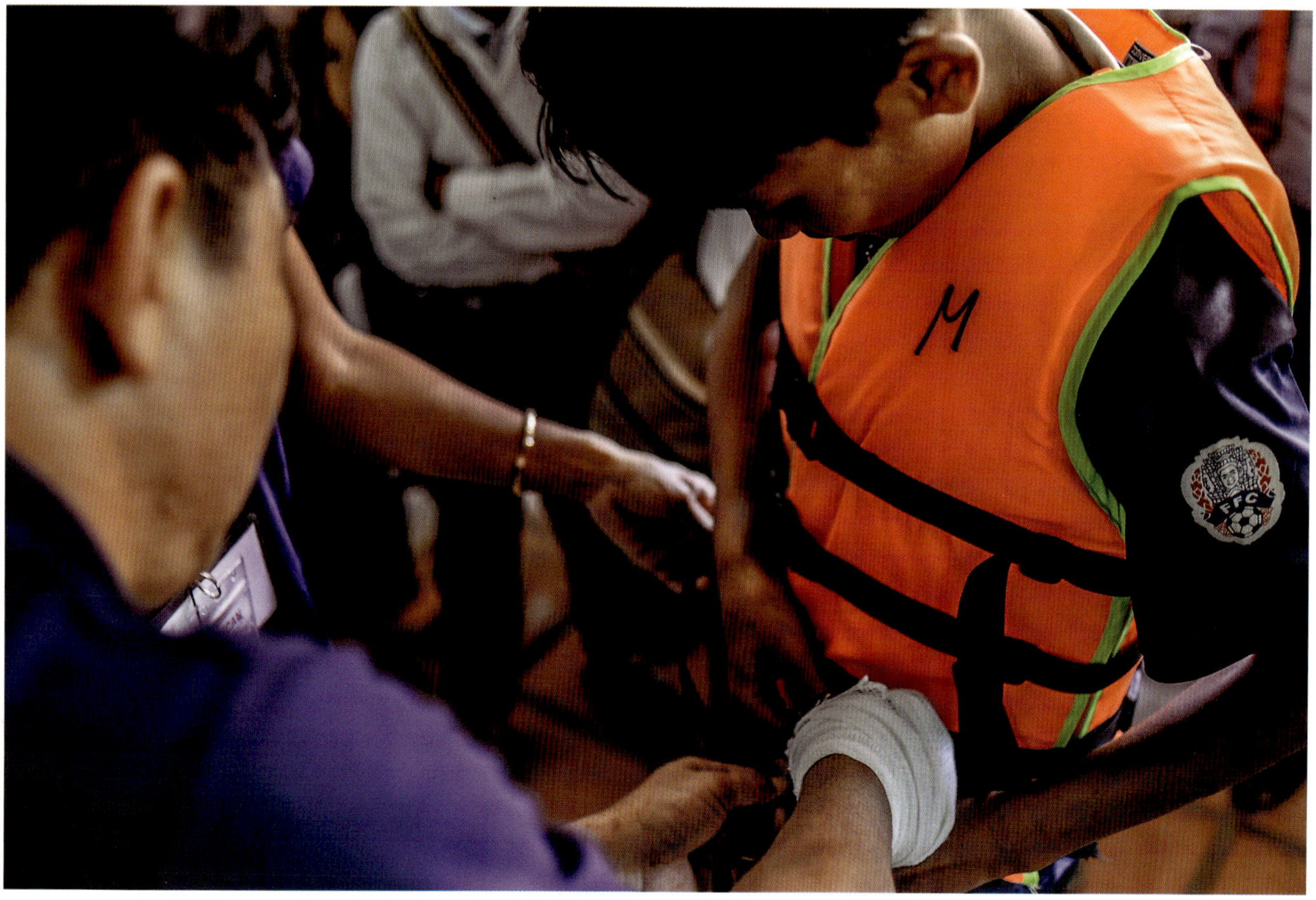

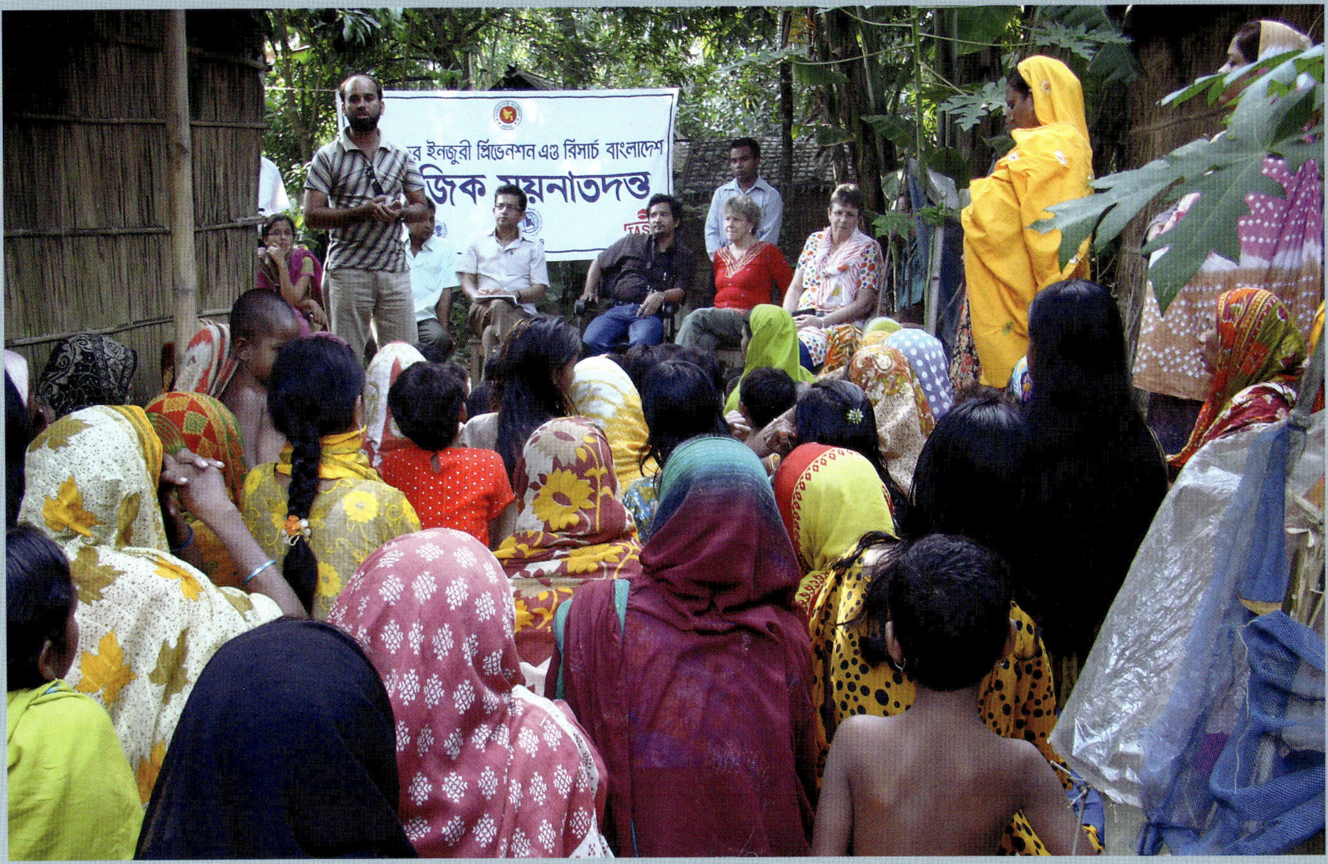

Case studies

Decreasing drowning through community education, Arizona USA, and Bangladesh

After a massive community education effort in Arizona in 1989, fatal and non-fatal drownings had decreased by almost 50% across the state by 1990. Messages included the need for adult supervision and for increased general acceptance of barriers around swimming pools to complement supervision. Prevention groups worked closely and in coalition with the mass media (newspapers, television and radio), hospitals and local businesses; provided information to elected officials; and participated in local, city and state public sessions focused on childhood drownings. Arizona also developed parental support groups for families of drowning and near-drowning victims *(108)*.

More recently, a drowning prevention package was formulated and piloted for 3 months in four rural communities in Bangladesh to assess its feasibility, acceptability and sustainability. Increased supervision of children, raising awareness of water safety and educating the community on safe rescue and resuscitation skills were the three core components of the intervention package. The awareness raising component emphasized the importance of child supervision, removing indoor drowning hazards and protecting children from outdoor water bodies by creating barriers such as fencing around a pond or home, installing door barriers or using playpens. To create heightened public awareness of water safety, formation of village committees and conducting "courtyard" and "social autopsy"[13] meetings with communities were considered *(109)*. The scale of this package was insufficient to assess effectiveness for drowning prevention at population level, however such efforts can reveal important process measures, including obstacles to the implementation of such programmes, and thereby establish feasibility, acceptability and sustainability.

13 A social or courtyard autopsy involves relatives or those closely involved with the drowning incident being interviewed about the social, environmental, health and behaviour conditions surrounding the event, any drowning prevention procedures followed, the type and timing of the intervention, and any barriers encountered during the intervention.

3

Establish a national water safety (drowning prevention) plan

A national water safety (or drowning prevention) plan sets out the main principles, goals, objectives, actions and coordination mechanisms for reducing and preventing fatal and non-fatal drowning *(110)*. These plans (sometimes called strategies or policies) may focus on drowning generally – or if data, political and/or community pressure dictates, on a specific aspect of drowning, for example swimming pool drowning deaths.

While there is limited published literature reviewing or evaluating the effectiveness of existing national water safety plans, evaluations of plans in other public health or development areas – such as preventing child injury, improving road safety or strengthening disaster risk reduction – show that national plans can work.

Benefits of a national water safety plan

Developing, implementing and evaluating a national water safety plan helps to:

- identify priority areas of drowning risk;
- identify and align efforts of stakeholders, including those not yet engaged in the issue;
- identify and allocate resources to areas of greatest need;
- raise awareness at political, policy and community levels;
- inform research agendas, including identifying gaps in data and interventions;
- provide a platform to engage government and develop additional laws, policy and regulations.

Establish a national water safety plan

There is no single model or process that can be recommended, but planners are encouraged to consider the following seven steps that reflect those outlined in the *Global report on drowning.*

⇩ Step one

Assess the situation

National or cohort data should be examined to provide key features of drowning contexts, highest risk populations, and lessons learned in order to inform national plan priorities. Include assessment of any national injury, health or disaster risk reduction plans that may provide opportunities for integration (see Situational assessment).

See page 5

⇩ Step two

Establish leadership

Drowning is a multisectoral challenge, so a successful national water safety plan requires strong leadership, effective planning and widespread stakeholder support. Leadership models include those led by government; those led by NGOs; and those led in partnership by government, United Nations

(UN) agencies and NGOs, etc. When deciding on leadership, devise a plan for achieving (eventual) government endorsement (see step 6).

See page 87

Some low- and middle-income country contexts may require the planning process to be led by government ministries, supported by UN agencies. For example, Table 4 outlines the role of the Government of Viet Nam and key ministries in leading the Viet Nam Plan of Action for Child Drowning Prevention 2010–2015, which delegates responsibilities and key actions down to provincial level.

Step three

Identify stakeholders

See page 67

Stakeholder mapping should reflect the multisectoral nature of drowning prevention (see Promote multisectoral collaboration). The recent Canadian Drowning Prevention Plan took an inclusive approach to stakeholder mapping, consultation and engagement, using workshops to explore drowning prevention from all perspectives and elicit the likely acceptance of interventions. A welcome by-product of this has been the creation of similar processes at provincial and community levels. Focus groups have also been successfully used in Bangladesh to inform the development of community drowning prevention action plans.

In low- and middle-income contexts where drowning risk is evident but not yet a focus, there may be substantial benefits in engaging health, disaster risk reduction, and water and sanitation sectors. For example, the water development sector in Cambodia aims to strengthen existing and build new waterways principally for economic, agricultural and health development. Areas of overlapping interest are evident, and partnership in planning is likely to increase opportunities for drowning prevention.

A review of existing water safety plans shows there is no one-size-fits-all framework, so part of the planning process requires stakeholders to determine the framework that best suits their setting.

Step four

Define a framework

National plans benefit from an organizing framework to give them structure and enable them to explicitly lay out their vision, goals and principles. A review of existing water safety plans shows there is no one-size-fits-all framework, so part of the planning process requires stakeholders to determine the framework that best suits their setting.

The choice of framework should take into consideration the extent to which it can secure political and financial support for the plan, and to communicate clearly to all stakeholders (including the public) the plan's goals and objectives.

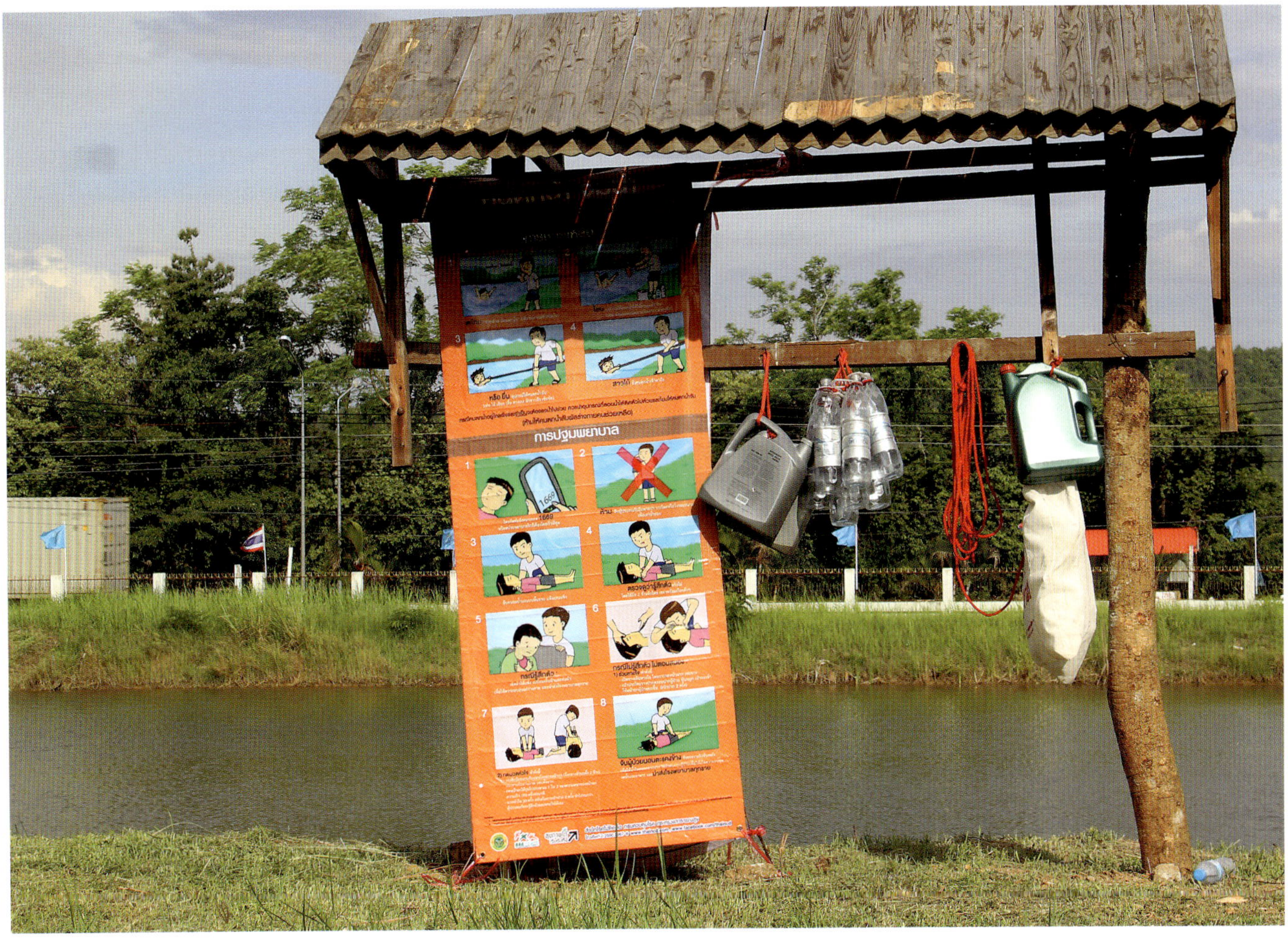

See page 87

Viet Nam (see Table 4) decided to frame its national plan around governmental department priorities and responsibilities. The Australian Water Safety Plan's organizing framework was rooted in goals and objectives agreed by stakeholders. The recently released UK Drowning Prevention Strategy 2016–2026 used analysis of drowning data to identify four strategic themes as its framework, corresponding to four main drivers of drowning events.

Step five

Set objectives and interventions

National plan objectives should be identified using information gathered during the assessment phase. They often address a country's priority drowning issues; need for data/ research; identification of interventions; and the importance of coordination and collaboration among partners. All national plans should promote the implementation of interventions based on best current evidence and explicitly assign responsibilities, coordination mechanisms and resource needs.

Step six

Gain government endorsement

Government endorsement is important and often difficult to obtain – but where gained, there is often evidence of solid action. Thailand's Child Drowning Action Plan *(111)*, led by the Ministry of Health, formed a child drowning committee, developed a swim skills and water safety policy and curriculum, and a requirement to link parental education on child drowning with the early childhood vaccination process.

Obtaining government endorsement can be helped by:

- involving stakeholders who can influence government, e.g. community leaders;
- providing regular updates on the development of the plan to heads of ministries;
- deciding a strategy at leadership designation stage to get government endorsement;
- being explicit about cost implications and how the plan will be funded;
- using the *Global report on drowning* to get sign off on the plan when it is ready.

In addition to the *Global report on drowning*, other catalysts for government involvement in developing plans include World Health Assembly Resolution WHA64.27 (2011) on child injury prevention, which specifically cited drowning as a major cause of child injury deaths. This Resolution urges Member States to prioritize the prevention of child injuries, including a call for the development of multisectoral policy and plans of action with realistic targets.

Step seven

Implementing and monitoring the plan

The national plan should be explicit when establishing objectives (see step 5) and allocating responsibility for achieving those objectives. Furthermore, monitoring the plan is both a matter of determining whether the specific objectives are being met and determining whether the plan's objectives need to be revised. There should be regular follow-up to monitor and report on how the plan is progressing to ensure ongoing engagement and strengthen collaboration. It should also be noted that the development process is as important as the plan itself, as it needs to promote collaboration, engagement, and build a coalition of partners willing to address drowning.

It should also be noted that the development process is as important as the plan itself, as it needs to promote collaboration, engagement, and build a coalition of partners willing to address drowning.

Drowning prevention plans in the wider context

Harness regional and global approaches

Regional plans provide a basis for strengthening capacity and focus on drowning as an issue across national governments, NGOs and the research sector. WHO has successfully promoted the development of regional and national injury prevention plans in the Western Pacific Region and the South-East Asia Region, including the Regional Action Plan for Violence and Injury Prevention in the Western Pacific 2016–2020 *(112)*.

Numerous efforts have been undertaken to focus attention and build capacity for the development of regional and national action plans. World Conferences on Drowning Prevention in 2011 and 2015, as well as numerous regional, national and stakeholder planning workshops have been conducted in partnership with NGOs, WHO, UNICEF and governments in the South-East Asia Region and the Western Pacific Region. More recently these have sought to understand and make recommendations in response to the *Global report on drowning* key actions.

Integrating drowning prevention into other sectoral plans

See page 67

The multisectoral nature of drowning prevention lends itself to integration with plans developed and implemented in other development sectors (see Promote multisectoral collaboration). Some examples of sectoral plans which have the potential to reduce drowning include those focused on disaster risk reduction at national, provincial and community levels; maritime safety plans of action; and plans to strengthen public health systems. Effective policy advocacy is needed to ensure the integration of drowning into such plans.

Table 4: Two approaches to developing a national water safety plan

Process	Australian Water Safety Strategy 2012–2015	Viet Nam Plan of Action for Child Drowning Prevention 2010–2015
Phase 1		
Assess the situation	Analysis of fatal drowning data drawn from coronial, police, media and NGO records.	Extensive analysis of drowning data resulted in the identification of 15 high-drowning provinces.
Raise awareness	Strategy is second iteration of a plan to reduce drowning by 50% by 2020.	Extensive use of publications and presentations in the context of the Viet Nam Child Injury Action Plan.
Identify leadership and foster political commitment	Led by Australian Water Safety Council (AWSC), made up principally of water safety focused NGOs.	Inter-ministerial Panel on Child Drowning convened and led by Ministry of Labour, Invalid and Social Affairs (MOLISA).
Involve stakeholders and create ownership	Participatory evaluation, redrafting and endorsement process implemented.	Engagement of key ministries and provincial representatives. Support provided by UN agencies WHO and UNICEF, and NGOs.
Phase 2		
Define a framework	Framework of goals focusing on key areas of risk; high-drowning-rate life stages, environments and activities.	Structured around ministerial responsibilities, and known evidence-based interventions.
Set objectives and select interventions	Objectives and interventions, including identifying research gaps, set across goals relating to: children; young people aged 15–24; people aged over 55 years; inland waterways; surf beaches; aquatic industry; alcohol and drugs; watercraft; high-risk populations; disaster and extreme weather.	Objectives and actions set in relation to: building local capacity; strengthening communication and public education; building models for a child-safe community and home; improving swimming and water safety teaching; tightening law, sanctions and regulations; mobilizing workforce for child protection; improving reporting, warning and first aid systems.
Ensure that the plan leads to action	Model involves AWSC members and state jurisdictions aligning their efforts to the plan.	Progress monitored via 6-monthly implementation review workshops. Vertical coordination of ministries into local provincial authorities.
Phase 3		
Stakeholder approval	Approved by AWSC.	Plan approved by inter-ministerial panel.
Government approval	Launched by representative of government, referred to in policy but not enshrined in legislation.	All agencies and provinces signed off on commitment to implementation activities.
State endorsement		Plan supported by Prime Minister in declaration.

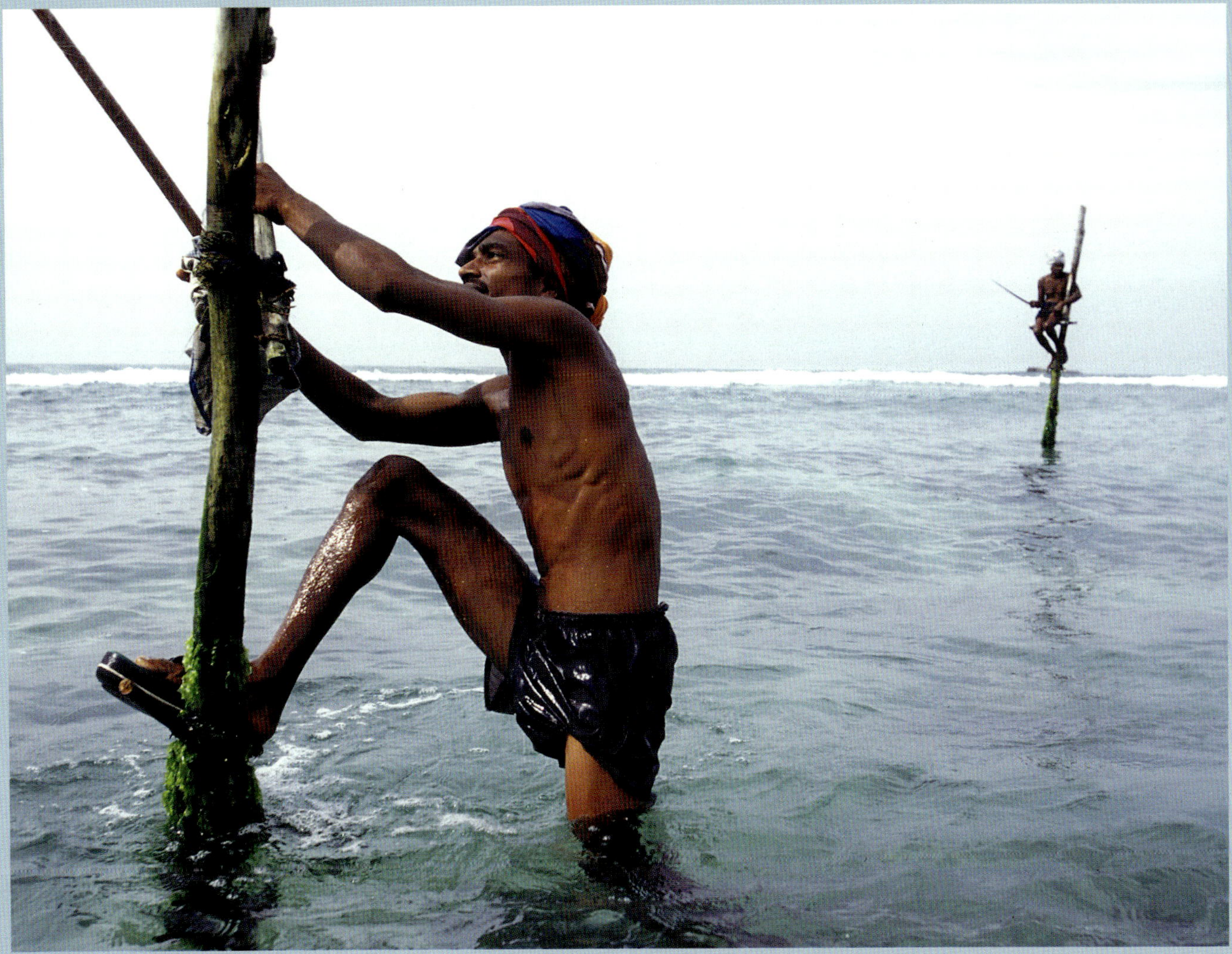

Case study
Drowning Prevention and Water Safety Plan, Sri Lanka

Sri Lanka's Drowning Prevention and Water Safety Plan *(113)* was based on a comprehensive situational assessment and stakeholder engagement. This arose from a WHO-supported research project to identify the patterns of drowning – the second leading cause of accidental death in Sri Lanka.

A data collection and analysis of drowning cases between 2004 and 2009 was conducted. The study identified risk factors for drowning; daily living such as bathing, working in agriculture or in construction, and recreational activities. Adults aged 25–44 years were at greatest risk, and males were four times more likely to drown than females. Alcohol consumption, lack of lifejacket use on boats, poor supervision practices, flooding during monsoon and unprotected wells and open reservoirs were identified as contributing factors.

Uniquely, the plan combines a focus on reducing drowning with the development of tourism, use of natural assets and increased employment opportunities. The plan has eight key strategies, and includes responsibilities for implementation by government, NGOs, external partners and the business sector under the guidance of the National Drowning Prevention and Water Safety Council *(113)*.

4

Research: advance drowning prevention through data collection and well-designed studies

Drowning is a leading, preventable and largely overlooked killer. To change this, data collection systems need to be improved, and in some cases established. In addition, well-designed studies are needed to advance drowning prevention through improved understanding of risk factors and the effectiveness of interventions – be they related to safe places for children, barriers, swim skills, boating and shipping regulation, flood resilience or safe rescue and resuscitation.

Benefits of research and advancing drowning prevention through data collection and well-designed studies

Well-designed research – both quantitative and qualitative – enables the best possible programmes to be developed, modified and monitored, and programme outcomes to be assessed *(114)*. It also allows programmes to be tailored to local contexts, and increases programme visibility among different audiences *(115)*.

What type of research is needed in the drowning prevention field?

Both quantitative and qualitative studies are needed to advance drowning prevention. It is beyond the scope of this resource guide to provide a comprehensive outline of how research should be carried out, but nonetheless, the type of research needed will likely depend on the level of attention currently given to the issue of drowning in a given setting – for example:

- where drowning is low or not on the public agenda, the first research step is analysing any existing data and improving data collection (see step 1);
- where the intention to address drowning based on data exists, but stakeholders are unsure of what to do and where, research to identify risk factors is likely the most relevant next step (see step 2);
- where interventions to prevent drowning are being implemented, research on their implementation and effectiveness is the most relevant next step (see step 3).

Based on which of these broad categories applies most closely, policy-makers and those concerned with drowning prevention should decide what type of research is most relevant. If they lack the relevant capacity to undertake it themselves, they can commission those that do.

⇩ Step one

Analyse existing data and improve data collection

Data collection systems – ongoing surveillance or periodic surveys – underpin much of what is known about drowning. In many settings, analysis of such data is an essential first step to preventing drowning as it can establish the scale of the problem and who is at risk. It also allows prioritization – determining where and what type of drowning prevention intervention is needed.

Where data are non-existent or of poor quality (particularly in low- and middle-income countries with weak or absent surveillance systems), steps should be taken to improve completeness, timeliness and accuracy for national systems – though this need not necessarily be addressed at a national level. A balance has to be struck between implementing drowning prevention interventions and establishing and refining national surveillance systems. Waiting for a fully functioning national surveillance system before implementing drowning prevention efforts means they may never start.

WHO's *Injury Surveillance Guidelines and the Fatal injury surveillance in mortuaries and hospitals guideline (116)* may be referred to for guidance on how to design, establish and maintain surveillance systems *(117)*. The addition of simple questions to routine data collections would potentially be effective in determining location (type of body of water) and activity at the time of submersion, and lead to targeted prevention strategies. If surveillance systems are weak, alternative methods can be used, including the following:

- **Community surveys** involving household interviews. These can provide detailed information on drowning and non-fatal drowning, and those done at different times can be used to monitor trends. While it should be noted that large samples are needed for such surveys, this should not be seen as a deterrent to carrying out the survey. Community surveys in South-East Asia have revealed the scale of the drowning problem and its role as a leading cause of death *(28)*. WHO's *Guidelines for conducting community surveys* can be referred to for developing a standardized tool for systematic collection of data, obtaining representative samples and using tools in the field *(118)*.
- **Verbal autopsies** (where circumstances surrounding deaths are described, allowing investigators to categorize deaths by likely cause) can be used to provide more detailed case studies of drowning events *(119)*.
- **Media reports** – while this form of data collection can be biased towards particular types of drowning and overlook drownings that happen away from the population, it can be a low-cost tool to collect drowning statistics *(120–122)*. Starting with the media allows you to understand what the community thinks about drowning and its risks, can provide rich data surrounding the circumstance of particular events, and helps develop appropriate strategies for reported cases.

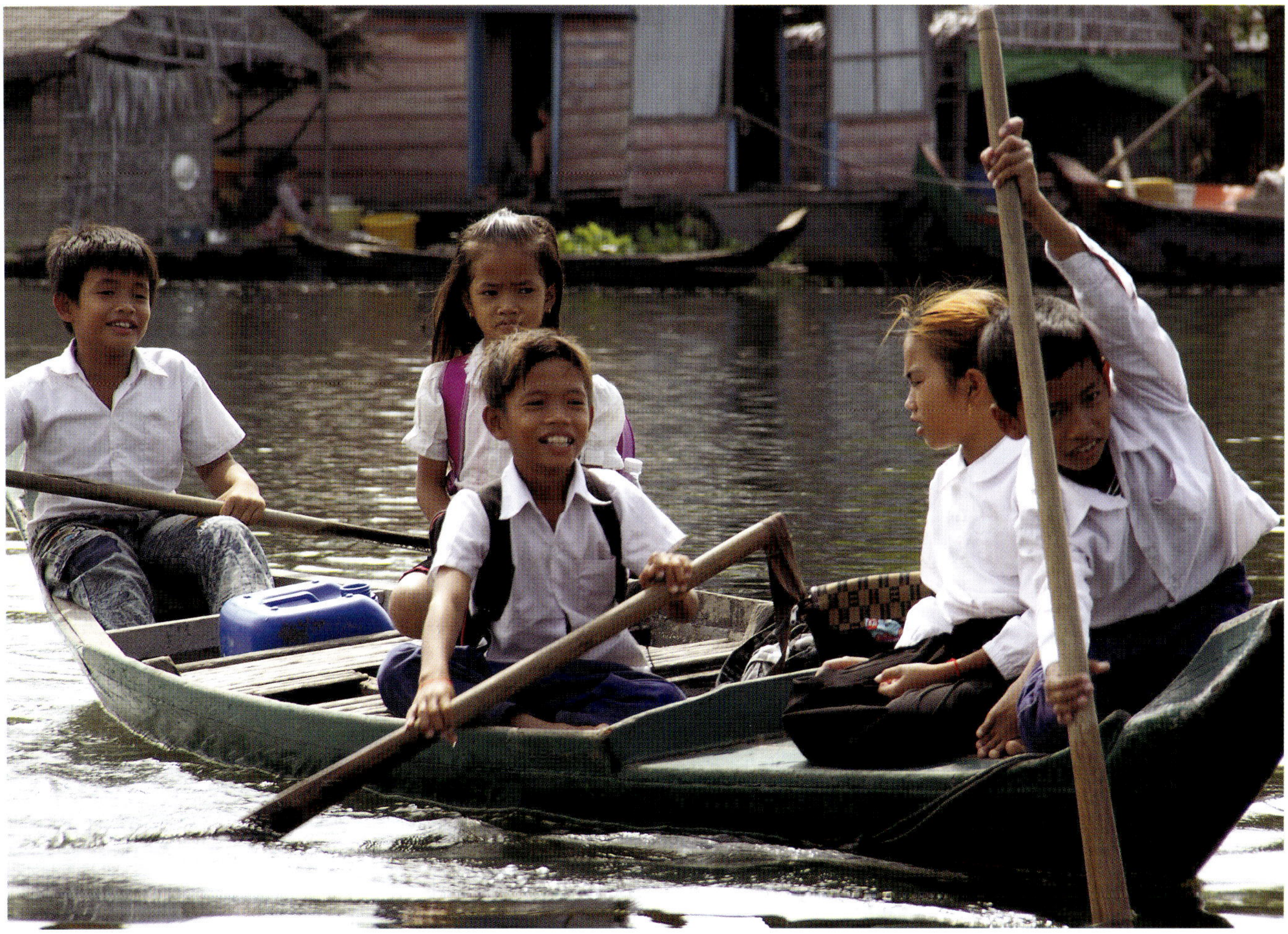

Understanding drowning circumstances allows researchers to identify risk factors for drowning, which in turn improves understanding of possible preventive actions.

⇩ Step two

Identify risk factors

Understanding drowning circumstances allows researchers to identify risk factors for drowning, which in turn improves understanding of possible preventive actions. Quantitative methods can be very helpful in establishing risk factors and risk groups within a population. Often initial findings from quantitative methods are better understood through the use of qualitative methods, such as focus groups and in-depth interviews with stakeholders. These include the following:

- **Community surveys** (such as those used in South-East Asia *(28)* as described above) provide a wealth of risk factor information such as: age groups or sex most at risk; occupational or activity risks; types of water bodies posing the greatest risk; and the importance of supervising children.
- **Research using qualitative methods, such as knowledge, attitudes and practice surveys.** These can provide valuable additional detail on key issues, including understanding of risk factors such as parents' perception of their own swimming ability and that of their children; socio-cultural barriers; or perceptions of the protective value of lifejackets, etc. Deeper understanding of these issues can help refine and improve the effectiveness of interventions, suggesting

ways to overcome barriers to implementation, and help identify risk factors or risk groups requiring a particular programmatic focus. For example, children with epilepsy and other seizure disorders have an increased risk of drowning.

- **Descriptive studies from surveillance data**, particularly where enhanced by a narrative on drowning circumstances *(123)*,[14] or studies of exposure to water hazards provide information on contributing factors and inform priority settings for interventions.
- **Key informant interviews** provide information on potential risk factors.

The evidence base for effective interventions to prevent drowning in low-income settings is emerging but small. This means implementers in these settings should make every effort to incorporate a research component in their programme design.

⇩ Step three

Research to improve understanding of intervention effectiveness and implementation

A number of literature reviews *(8, 26, 124, 125)* on drowning prevention reveal that effective interventions include engineering, environmental, legislative/regulatory and educational measures, and drowning management. Much of what is known about the effectiveness of these approaches comes from high-income countries, leaving gaps in our understanding of whether and how these can be adapted for low-income settings.

The evidence base for effective interventions to prevent drowning in low-income settings is emerging but small. This means implementers in these settings should make every effort to incorporate a research component in their programme design (regardless of scale), with the objective of conducting a well-designed study or studies to add to the peer-reviewed literature. A range of potentially relevant tools for implementation research are discussed in WHO's *Implementation research in health: a practical guide (126)*. These include:

- **cost data research**, which can help make the case for preventive interventions. While detailed guidance is beyond the scope of this publication, many examples of cost data research can be drawn upon, including some that have taken place in the drowning prevention area *(4)*. Such information is extremely helpful to stimulate the interest of drowning prevention policy-makers, and much more cost data are needed in the drowning prevention area.

14 A newly published "drowning timeline" that breaks the drowning process into pre-event, event and post-event presents a tool for improved drowning data collection that can contribute to a better understanding of the process to effectively prevent, react and mitigate it. It can also help prioritize the deployment of resources *(123)*.

- **qualitative studies,** which can be used to assess the appropriateness and effectiveness of interventions in particular settings by finding out how people in the potential intervention settings view the "problem" to be addressed. Qualitative research can also uncover why interventions fail.
- **Identifying good practice**: when an intervention is being implemented in a particular setting it is helpful to identify which factors may help or hinder. For example, this could include rapid turnover of staff, the need for training in multi-agency working, the role of a champion, etc. There is the need to identify what has worked and what has not worked and to summarize these issues. In this way good practices for replicating the intervention in other settings can be captured.

Additional methods include:

- **intermediate or impact measurement** which is indicative (and explanatory) of a proven relationship between the intermediate measure and drowning prevention (e.g. children taught to swim, small vessel occupants wearing lifejackets, wells covered etc.);
- **quasi-experimental studies** (essentially "before and after studies") where matched controls (e.g. comparison communities) are used to determine whether the intervention was effective beyond the effects of general community programmes and trends.

A framework for effective implementation of drowning interventions has been developed and is being tested in the Saving of Lives from Drowning (SoLiD) Project in Bangladesh *(9)*. The framework comprises four phases: planning, engaging, executing and evaluating. This framework is a useful tool that has the potential to be adapted to drowning and other injury prevention programmes in low- and middle-income settings *(9)*.

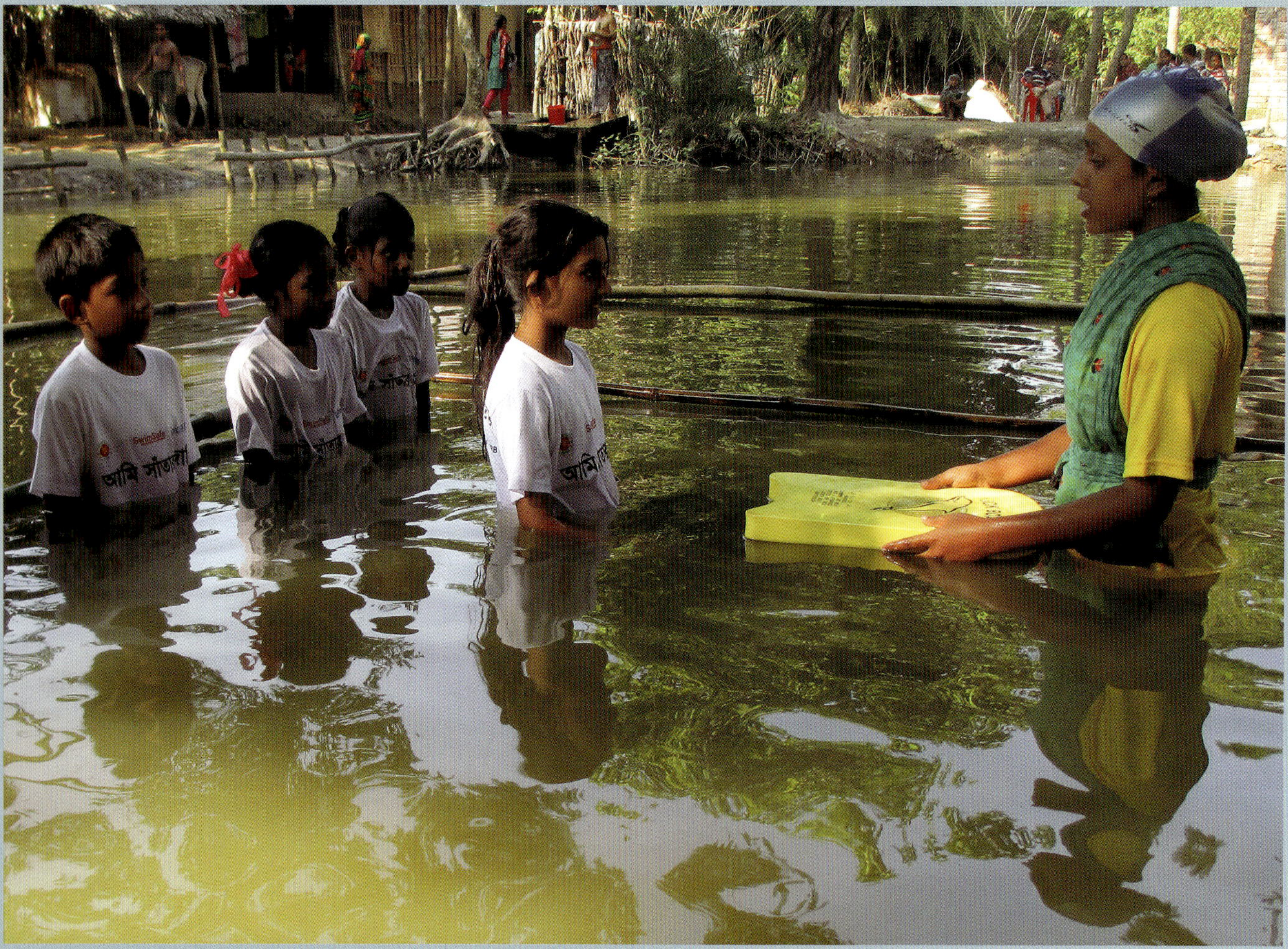

Case study
Stages in the development of the SwimSafe Programme in different settings, using the public health approach, Bangladesh

Surveillance

A large-scale community-based survey, the Bangladesh Health and Injury Survey (BHIS), found than drowning dominated the overall spectrum of child injury deaths *(33)*. It was the single leading cause of deaths in children aged 1–17 years, and claimed more victims than pneumonia, malnutrition and diarrhoea combined *(33)*.

Identifying risk factors

BHIS also identified different drowning dangers at different ages, and this information was supplemented by focus groups in local communities and consultation with stakeholders. One high-risk group identified was school-age children drowning away from home, where they swim alone or with peers who do not have swimming, rescue or resuscitation skills *(33)*.

Developing and evaluating interventions

In Bangladesh, the Prevention of Child Injury through Social Intervention and Education (PRECISE) Programme was developed to address various causal factors in drowning. A swimming skills programme called SwimSafe – a structured community based programme of swimming and water safety skills – focused on children aged 4–10 years. The SwimSafe curriculum – which teaches 18–22 basic swimming and water survival skills in up to 20 lessons – was delivered by trained local swimming instructors in village ponds *(34)*.

Implementing effective interventions

The delivery and content of the programme has evolved over time in Bangladesh, following extensive local consultation, illustrating the power of qualitative data. One evolution has been the increase in the number

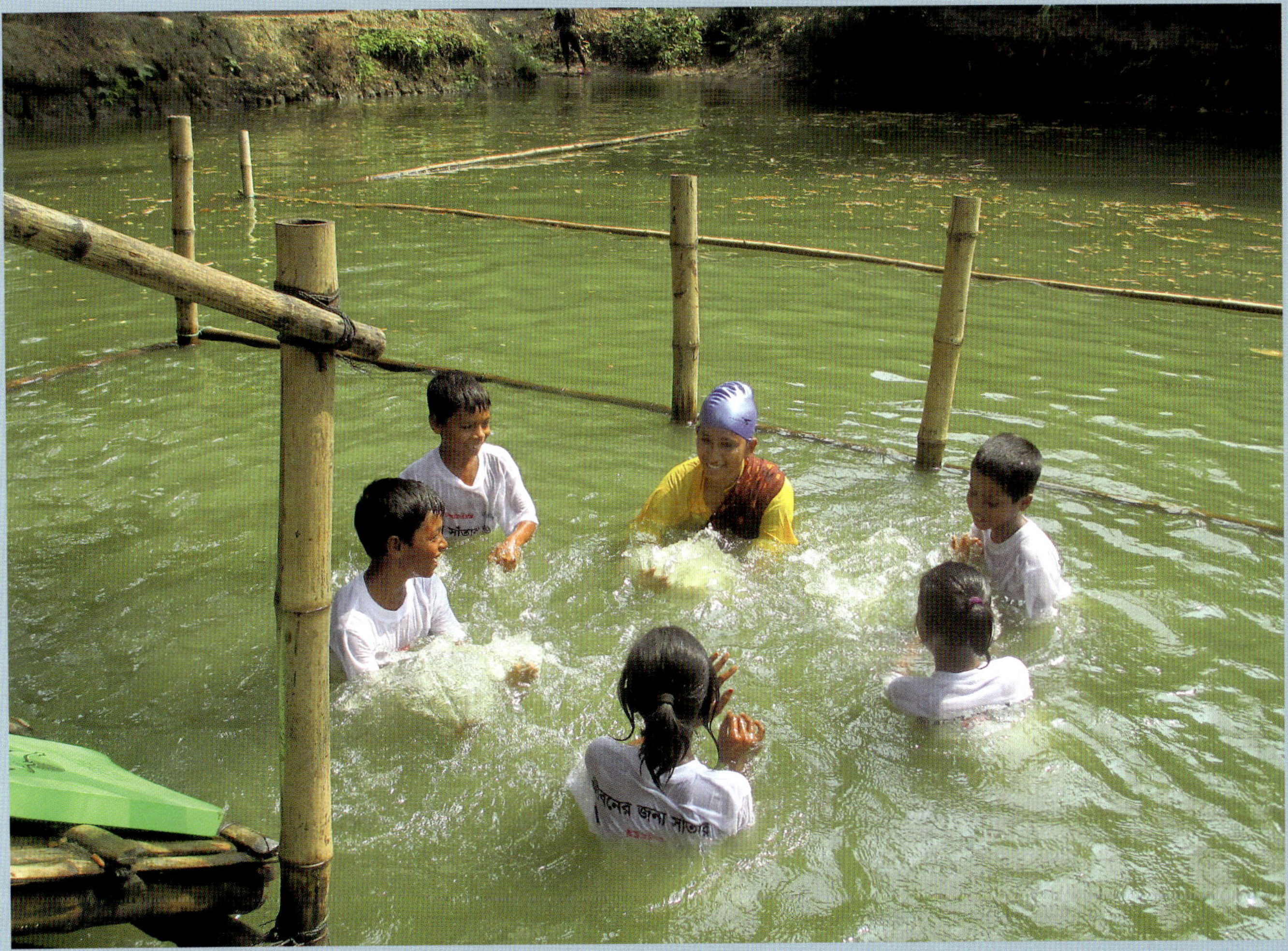

of female swimming instructors, and learning that local ponds can only be used at certain times of year in Bangladesh.

When the programme was modified for use in Viet Nam it was adapted to be a school-based initiative using portable pools, with school teachers providing instruction *(127)*. The programme targeted children aged 6–12 years and was taught over 20 lessons. CPR was introduced for children aged over 9 years. Consultation with stakeholders from the local community enabled the programme to be tailored to local environments and conditions. For example, in Viet Nam there was the acceptance of training children to swim in portable, above ground pools rather than adapting local ponds (as in Bangladesh). As the portable pools could be located adjacent to schools, school teachers could then be recruited more easily as swimming instructors. However, despite the programme being adapted, the main aim of the training programme has been retained and a staged approach used in the development of swimming skills.

Conclusion

Some settings will benefit from active cooperation by many sectors, while in others progress will rely on a much smaller number of actors. But one shared and common asset will always be the desire to act.

Drowning is a leading global killer, particularly among children and young adults. It is preventable but neglected relative to its impact on families, communities and livelihoods.

This guide provides concrete support to drowning prevention practitioners implementing drowning prevention interventions. Drowning prevention can begin with the effective implementation of a single intervention (though multiple interventions implemented in tandem, supported by all relevant strategies, will strengthen impact), or it may involve a more wide-ranging set of interventions that are implemented in the context of a much more comprehensive drowning prevention effort.

Different settings will have different drowning problems and levels of resources to tackle them. Some settings will benefit from active cooperation by many sectors, while in others progress will rely on a much smaller number of actors. But one shared and common asset will always be the desire to act.

Users of this guide may not be able to undertake all the measures it contains, but with commitment and determination to act, a start can be made. This guide provides the basis to translate the desire to act into concrete, targeted and evidence-based actions to prevent drowning and save lives.

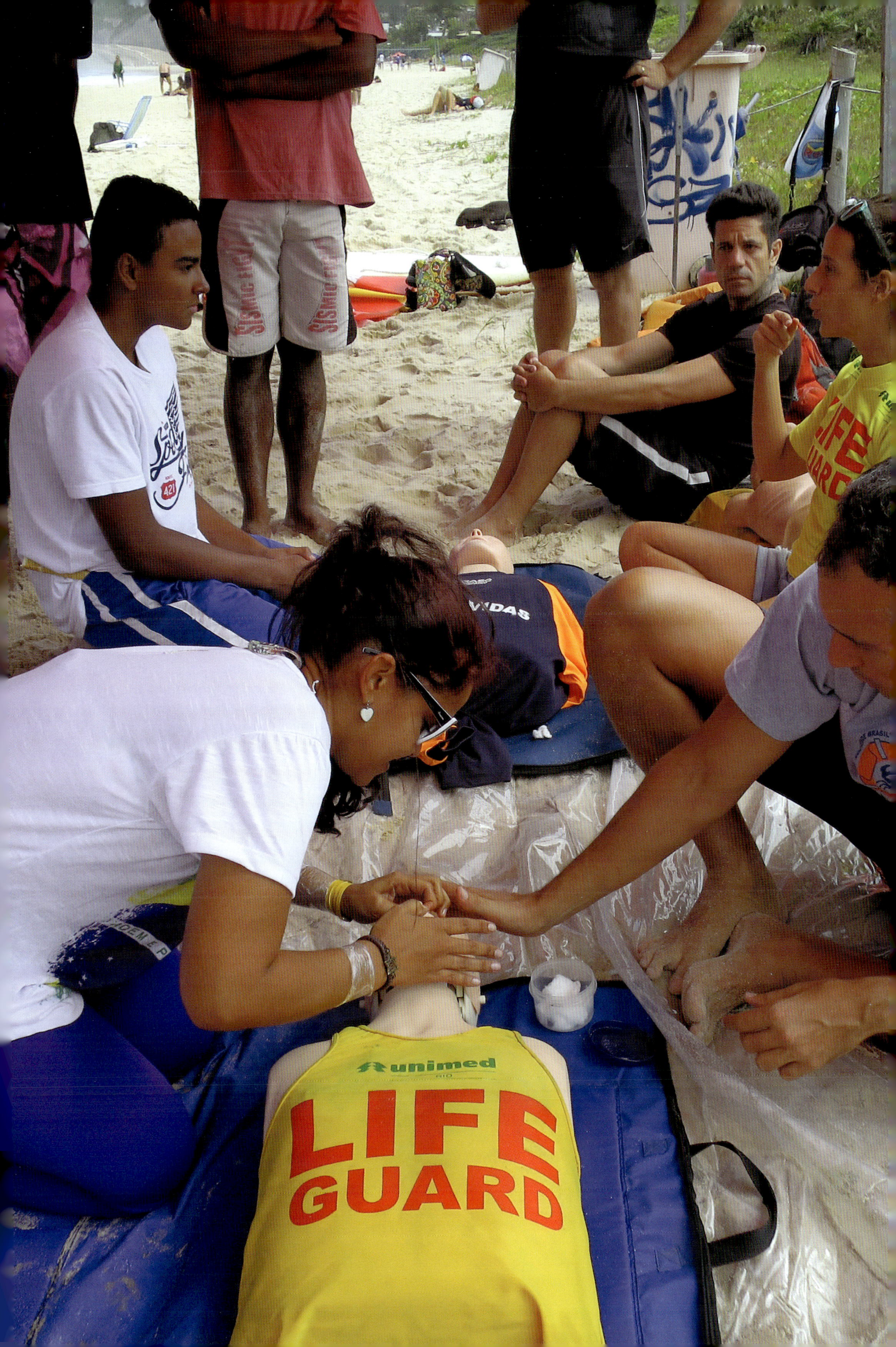
unimed
LIFE
GUARD

References

1
Global report on drowning: preventing a leading killer. Geneva: World Health Organization; 2014.

2
Guidelines for conducting community surveys on injuries and violence. Geneva: World Health Organization; 2004.

3
Mello-Jorge MH, Marques MB. Violent childhood deaths in Brazil. Bulletin of the Pan American Health Organization. 1985;19: 288–99.

4
Rahman F, Bose S, Linnan M et al. Cost-effectiveness of an injury and drowning prevention program in Bangladesh. Pediatrics. 2012;130(6):e1621–8.

5
Thompson DC et al. Pool fencing for preventing drowning in children. Cochrane Database of Systematic Reviews. 2000;(2):CD001047.

6
Depczynski J, Fragar L, Hawkins A, Stiller L. Safe play areas for prevention of young children drowning in farm dams. Australasian Journal of Early Childhood. 2009;34(3):50–58.

7
Iqbal A et al. Childhood mortality due to drowning in rural Matlab of Bangladesh: magnitude of the problem and proposed solutions. Journal of Health, Population and Nutrition. 2007;25(3):370–376.

8
Hyder AA, Alonge O, He S, Wadhwaniya S, Rahman F, Rahman A et al. A framework for addressing implementation gap in global drowning prevention interventions: experiences from Bangladesh. Journal of Health, Population and Nutrition. 2014;32(4):564–576.

9
Hyder AA, Alonge O, He S, Wadhwaniya S, Rahman F, Rahman A et al. Saving of children's Lives from Drowning project in Bangladesh. American Journal of Preventive Medicine. 2014;47(6):842–845.

10
Callaghan JA, Hyder AA, Khan R, Blum LS, Arifeen S, Baqui AH. Child supervision practices for drowning prevention in rural Bangladesh: a pilot study of supervision tools. Journal of Epidemiology and Community Health. 2010;64(7):645–647.

11
Islam I, Sharmin Salam S, Hoque DME, Sadeq-ur Rahman Q, Alonge O, Hyder AA, El Arifeen S. Preliminary findings on the utilization of playpens to prevent child drowining in rural Bangaldesh. Paper presented at World Conference on Drowning Prevention, Malaysia, 2015.

12
Bennett E, Linnan M. Physical barriers. In: Bierens JLM. Drowning: prevention, rescue, treatment. Second Edition. Berlin: Springer-Verlag; 2014.

13
Yeh S, Rochette LM, McKenzie LB, Smith GA. Injuries associated with cribs, playpens and bassinets among young children in the US, 1990–2008. Pediatrics. 2011;127(3):479–486.

14
Consumer Product Safety Commission, Safety Standard for Play Yards 2012 (https://www.cpsc.gov/Newsroom/News-Releases/2012/CPSC-Approves-New-Federal-Safety-Standard-for-Play-Yards1 accessed 5 November 2016).

15
Cordovil R, Barreiros F, Vieira F, Neto C. The efficacy of safety barriers for children: absolute efficacy, time to cross and action modes in children between 19 and 75 months. International Journal of Injury Control and Safety Promotion. 2009;16(3):143–151.

16
Full-size baby cribs and non-full-size baby cribs: safety standards; revocation of requirements; third party testing for certain children's products; final rules. Federal Register. 2010;75:248.

17
The safe nursery. A booklet to help avoid injuries from nursery furniture and equipment: buyer's guide. Washington, DC: U.S. Consumer Product Safety Commission; 1993.

18
Nixon JW, Pearn JH, Petrie GM. Childproof safety barriers: an ergonomic study to reduce child trauma due to environmental hazards. Journal of Paediatrics and Child Health. 1979;15(4):260–262.

19
Playpen Safety [website]. Ilinois, USA: American Academy of Pediatrics; 2015 (https://www.healthychildren.org/English/safety-prevention/at-home/Pages/Playpen-Safety.aspx, accessed 5 November 2016).

20
Deaths associated with playpens. Maryland, USA: U.S. Consumer Product Safety Commission; 2001 (http://www.cpsc.gov//PageFiles/108029/playpen.pdf, accessed 5 November 2016).

21
Guevarra J, Franklin R, Basilio J, Orbillo L, Go JJ. Child drowning prevention in the Philippines: the beginning of a conversation. International Journal of Injury Control and Safety Promotion. 2015;22:243–253.

22
Celis A. Home drowning among pre-school age Mexican children. Injury Prevention. 1997;3:252 256.

23
Ellis AA, Trent RB. Swimming pool drownings and near-drownings among California preschoolers. Public Health Reports. 1997;112(1):73–77.

24
Pearn JH, Nixon J, Franklin R, Wallis B. Safety legislation, public health policy and drowning prevention. International journal of injury control and safety promotion. 2008;15(2):122–123.

25
Stevenson MR, Miroslava R, Edgecombe D, Vickery K. Childhood drowning: barriers surrounding private swimming pools. Pediatrics. 2003;111(2):E115–119.

26
World report on child injury prevention. Geneva: World Health Organization; 2008.

27
WHO Fact Sheet on Drowning. Geneva: World Health Organization; 2014.

28
Linnan M, Rahman A, Scarr J, Reinten-Reynolds T, Linnan H, Rui-wei J et al. Child drowning: evidence for a newly recognized cause of child mortality in low- and middle-income countries and its prevention. Working Paper 2012–07, Special Series on Child Injury No. 2. Florence: UNICEF Office of Research; 2012.

29
Linnan M, Giersing M, Cox R, Linnan H, Williams MK, Voumard C, Hatfield R. Child mortality and injury in Asia: an overview. Innocenti Working Paper 2007–04, Special Series on Child Injury No. 1. Florence: UNICEF Innocenti Research Centre; 2007.

30
Stallman R, Moran K, Brenner RA, Rahman A. Swimming and water survival competence. Drowning. In: Bierens JLM. Drowning: prevention, rescue, treatment. Second Edition. Berlin: Springer-Verlag; 2014.

31
Brenner RA, Taneja GS, Haynie DL, Trumble AC, Qian C, Klinger RM, Klevanoff MA. Association between swimming lessons and drowning in childhood: a case-control study. Archives of Pediatrics & Adolescent Medicine. 2009;163(3):203–10.

32
Yang L, Nong QQ, Li CL, Feng QM, Lo SK. Risk factors for childhood drowning in rural regions of a developing country: a case-control study. Injury Prevention. 2007;13:178–182.

33
Rahman A, Rahman F, Shafinaz S, Linnan M. Bangladesh Health and Injury Survey: report on children. Dhaka: UNICEF; 2005:54.

34
Rahman F, Bose S, Linnan M, Rahman A, Mashreky S, Haaland B. Cost effectiveness of an injury and drowning prevention program in Bangladesh. Pediatrics. 2012;130(6):e1621-8. doi: 10.1542/peds.2012-0757.

35
SwimSafe [website] (www.swimsafe.org, accessed 5 November 2016).

36
Mecrow T, Linnan M, Rahman A, Scarr J, Mashreky SR, Talab A et al. Does teaching children to swim increase exposure or risk-taking when in the water? Emerging evidence from Bangladesh. Injury Prevention. 2015;21:185-188. doi:10.1136/injuryprev-2013-041053.

37
Mecrow T, Rahman A, Linnan M, Scarr J, Mashreky SR, Talab A et al. Children reporting rescuing other children drowning in rural Bangladesh: a descriptive study. Injury Prevention. 2015;21:185–188 doi:10.1136/injuryprev-2013-041053.

38
Making development sustainable: the future of disaster risk management. Global assessment report on disaster risk reduction. Geneva: United Nations Office for Disaster Risk Reduction; 2015.

39
Jonkman SN, Kelman I. An analysis of the causes and circumstances of flood disaster deaths. Disasters. 2005;29:75–97.

40
Haynes K, Coates L, Leigh R, Handmer J, Whittaker J, Gissing A et al. "Shelter-in-place" vs. evacuation in flash floods. Environmental Hazards. 2009;8:291–303.

41
Jonkman S. Loss of life due to floods: General overview. In: Bierens JLM. Drowning: prevention, rescue, treatment. Second Edition. Berlin: Springer-Verlag; 2014.

42
Diakakis M, Deligiannakis G. Flood fatalities in Greece: 1970–2010. Journal of Flood Risk Management. 2015. doi: 10.1111/jfr3.12166.

43
Jonkman SN, Maaskant B, Boyd E, Levitan ML. Loss of life caused by the flooding of New Orleans after Hurricane Katrina: analysis of the relationship between flood characteristics and mortality. Risk Analysis. 2009;29:676–698.

44
Climate Change 2014: Synthesis Report. Contribution of Working Groups I, II and III to the Fifth Assessment Report of the Intergovernmental Panel on Climate Change. Geneva: Intergovernmental Panel on Climate Change; 2014.

45
Hirabayashi Y, Mahendran R, Koirala S, Konoshima L, Yamazaki D, Watanabe S et al. Global flood risk under climate change. Nature Climate Change. 2013;3:816–821.

46
Hallegatte S, Green C, Nicholls RJ, Corfee-Morlot J. Future flood losses in major coastal cities. Nature Climate Change. 2013;3:802–806.

47
Chan FKS, Mitchell G, Adekola O, Mcdonald A. Flood risk in Asia's urban mega-deltas: drivers, impacts and response. Environment and Urbanization Asia. 2012;3:41–61.

48
Syvitski JP, Kettner AJ, Overeem I, Hutton EW, Hannon MT, Brakenridge GR et al. Sinking deltas due to human activities. Nature Geoscience. 2009;2: 681–686.

49
Global report on drowning. Geneva: World Health Organization; 2014.

50
Sendai Framework for Disaster Risk Reduction 2015–2030. Geneva: UNISDR; 2015.

51
Sobrasa and ILS Americas' Flood drowning prevention cartoon (https://www.youtube.com/watch?v=g6XLRu-bloc accessed 5 November 2016).

52
Daellenbach K, Waugh DW, Smith K. Community response planning. Victoria, Australia: Victoria University of Wellington; 2015.

53
Benson D, Lorenzoni I, Cook H. Evaluating social learning in England flood risk management: an 'individual-community interaction' perspective. Environmental Science & Policy. 2016;55:326–334.

54
Van Den Honert RC, Mcaneney J. The 2011 Brisbane floods: causes, impacts and implications. Water. 2011;3:1149–1173.

55
Managing the floodplain: a guide to best practice in flood risk management in Australia. Canberra, Australia: Attorney-General's Department; 2013.

56
Janssen SK, Van Tatenhove JP, Otter HS, Mol AP. Greening flood protection: an Interactive knowledge arrangement perspective. Journal of Environmental Policy & Planning. 2015;17:309–331.

57
Temmerman S, Meire P, Bouma TJ, Herman PMJ, Ysebaert T, De Vriend HJ. Ecosystem-based coastal defence in the face of global change. Nature. 2013;504:79–83.

58
Barbier EB. Valuing the storm protection service of estuarine and coastal ecosystems. Ecosystem Services. 2015;11:32–38.

59
Jones HP, Hole DG, Zavaleta ES. Harnessing nature to help people adapt to climate change. Nature Climate Change. 2012;2:504–509.

60
Dixon SJ, Sear DA, Odoni NA, Sykes T, Lane SN. The effects of river restoration on catchment scale flood risk and flood hydrology. Earth Surface Processes and Landforms. 2016;41:997–1008. doi:10.1002/esp.3919.

61
Managing the risks of extreme events and disasters to advance climate change adaptation. A special report of working groups I and II of the Intergovernmental Panel on Climate Change. Cambridge, UK: Cambridge University Press; 2012.

62
Hossain M, Mani KK, Sidik SM, Hayati KS, Rahman AK. Socio-demographic, environmental and caring risk factors for childhood drowning deaths in Bangladesh. Biomed Central Pediatrics. 2015;15:114. doi: 10.1186/s12887-015-0431-7.

63
Venema AM, Groothoff JW, Bierens JJ. The role of bystanders during rescue and resuscitation of drowning victims. Resuscitation, 2010;81:434–9.

64
Franklin RC, Pearn JH. Drowning for Love. The Aquatic-Victim-Instead-of-Rescuer (AVIR) Syndrome: Drowning fatalities involving those attempting to rescue a child. Journal of Paediatrics and Child Health. 2011;47(1–2):44–47.

65
Rahman A, Mecrow T, Rahman Mashreky S, Rahman F, Nusrat N, Khanama, M, Scarr J. Feasibility of a first responder programme in rural Bangladesh. Resuscitation. 2014;85:1088–1092.

66
Tate R, Quan L. Cultural aspects of rescue and resuscitation of drowning victims. In: Bierens J. Drowning: prevention, rescue, treatment. Second Edition. Berlin: Springer-Verlag; 2014:399–403

67
Mecrow T, Suvanprakorn A. Water safety skills and knowledge in the low-resource environment. In: Bierens JLM. Drowning: prevention, rescue, treatment. Second Edition. Berlin: Springer-Verlag; 2014:215–223.

68
Mecrow TS, Rahman A, Mashreky SR, Rahman F, Nusrat N, Scarr J, Linnan M. Willingness to administer mouth-to-mouth ventilation in a first response program in rural Bangladesh. Biomedical Central International Health and Human Rights. 2015;15:19. doi: 10.1186/s12914-015-0057-8.

69
Husum H, Gilbert M, Wisborg T. Training pre-hospital trauma care in low-income countries: the "village university" experience. Medical Teacher. 2003;25(2):142–8.

70
López-Herce J, Urbano J, Carrillo A, Matamoros M. Resuscitation training in developing countries: importance of a stable program of formation of instructors. Resuscitation. 2011;82(6):780.

71
European Resuscitation Council [website] (https://www.erc.edu, accessed 5 November 2016).

72
American Heart Association Guidelines Update for Cardiopulmonary Resuscitation and Emergency Cardiovascular Care [website]. Texas, USA: American Heart Association; 2015 (https://eccguidelines.heart.org/index.php/circulation/cpr-ecc-guidelines-2/, accessed 5 November 2016).

73
International first aid and resuscitation guidelines 2016. Geneva: International Federation of Red Cross and Red Crescent Societies; 2016 (http://www.ifrc.org/Global/Publications/Health/First-Aid-2016-Guidelines_EN.pdf, accessed 5 November 2016).

74
International Life Saving Federation [website] (http://www.ilsf.org/about/position-statements, accessed 5 November 2016).

75
IMRF Rescue Boat Guidelines. Aberdeen, UK: International Maritime Rescue; 2016 (http://international-maritime-rescue.org/homerbg, accessed 5 November 2016).

76
Truhlá A, Deakin CD, Soar J, Khalifa GE, Alfonzo A, Bierens JJ et al. Cardiac arrest in special circumstances. European Resuscitation Council Guidelines for Resuscitation, 2015: Section 4. Resuscitation. 2015;95:148–201.

77
Meaney PA, Topjian AA, Chandler HK, Botha M, Soar J, Berg RA, Nadkarni VM. Resuscitation training in developing countries: a systematic review. Resuscitation. 2010;81(11):1462–72.

78
Szpilman D. Near-drowning and drowning classification: a proposal to stratify mortality based on the analysis of 1831 cases. Chest. 1997;112(3):660–5.

79
European Resuscitation Council Guidelines for Resuscitation 2015: Section 10. Education and implementation of resuscitation [website] (http://ercguidelines.elsevierresource.com/european-resuscitation-council-guidelines-resuscitation-2015-section-10-education-and-implementation/fulltext, accessed 5 November 2016).

80
De Vries W, Bierens JJ. Instructor retraining and poster retraining are equally effective for the retention of BLS and AED skills of lifeguards. European Journal of Emergency Medicine. 2010;17(3):150–7.

81
Leavy JE, Crawford G, Portsmouth L, Jancey J, Leaversuch F, Nimmo L et al. Recreational drowning prevention interventions for adults, 1990–2012: a review. Journal of Community Health. 2015;40(4):725–35.

82
Cassell E, Newstead S. Did compulsory wear regulations increase personal flotation device (PFD) use by boaters in small power recreational vessels? A before-after observational study conducted in Victoria, Australia. Injury Prevention. 2015;21(1): 15–22.

83
Bugeja L, Cassell E et al. The effectiveness of the 2005 compulsory personal flotation device (PFD) wearing regulations in reducing drowning deaths among recreational boaters in Victoria, Australia. Injury Prevention. 2014;20(6):387–92.

84
Mangione T, Chow W. Changing lifejacket wearing behavior: an evaluation of two approaches. Journal of Public Health Policy. 2014;35(2):204–18.

85
Golden AS, Weisbrod RE. Trends, causal analysis, and recommendations from 14 years of ferry accidents. Journal of Public Transportation. 2016;19:1.

86
First five 3D printed NCAR weather stations installed in Zambia. 3D printer and 3D printing news [website] (http://www.3ders.org/articles/20160604-first-five-3d-printed-ncar-weather-stations-installed-in-zambia.html, accessed 5 November 2016).

87
Atmos News [website]. 3d printers promise affordable weather stations for the developing world (http://www2.ucar.edu/atmosnews/in-brief/16353/3d-printers-promise-affordable-weather-stations-developing-world, accessed 5 November 2016).

88
NOAA Satellite and information service [website] (http://www.nesdis.noaa.gov /GOES-R/pdf/goes-r-l-30-press- release_oct6.pdf, accessed 5 November 2016).

89
Ahmed D. Innovative E-Government best practices in early warning system for disaster risk management: Bangladesh experience. Dakha: Government of Bangladesh, Department of Disaster Management; (date unknown) (http://www.unosd.org/content/documents/1069EWS%20Dilder%20Ahmed%20revised.pdf, accessed 5 November 2016).

90
Early warning of disasters: facts and figures. SciDevNet [website]. (http://www.scidev.net/global/communication/feature/early-warning-of-disasters-facts-and-figures-1.html, accessed 5 November 2016).

91
List of IMO conventions. In: International Maritime Organization [website]. London: International Maritime Organization; 2016 (http://www.imo.org/en/About/Conventions/ListOfConventions/Pages/Default.aspx, accessed 5 November 2016).

92
Welch DJ. A small-scale vessel registration system for Pacific Island countries and territories. New Caledonia: Pacific Community; 2016.

93
Stempski S, Schiff M, Bennett E, Quan L. A case-control study of boat-related injuries and fatalities in Washington State. Injury Prevention. 2014;20: 232–237.

94
Smith GS, Keyl PM, Hadley JA, Bartley CL, Foss RD, Tolbert WG et al. Drinking and recreational boating fatalities: a population-based case-control study. JAMA. 2001;286:2974e80.

95
US Coastguard 2015 Recreational Boating Statistics. COMDTPUB P16754.29. Washington DC: US Department of Homeland Security; 2016.

96
Offences and penalties. In: Roads and Maritime [website]. New South Wales: Roads and Maritime; 2016 (http://www.rms.nsw.gov.au/maritime/safety-rules/offences-penalties.html, accessed 6 November 2016).

97
Kobusingye O, Tumwesigye NM, Magoola J, Atuyambe L, Olange O. Drowning among the lakeside fishing communities in Uganda: results of a community survey. International Journal of Injury Control and Safety Promotion. 2016;4:1–8.

98
Bugeja L, Cassell E, Brodie L, Walter S. The effectiveness of the 2005 compulsory personal flotation device (PFD) wearing regulations in reducing drowning deaths among recreational boaters in Victoria, Australia. Injury Prevention. 2014;20(6):387–92.

99
Cummings P, Mueller BA, Quan L. Association between wearing a personal floatation device and death by drowning among recreational boaters: a matched cohort analysis of United States Coast Guard data. Injury Prevention. 2011;17(3):156–9.

100
Chung C, Quan L, Bennett E, Kernic MA, Ebel BE. Informing policy on open water drowning prevention: an observational survey of lifejacket use in Washington State. Injury Prevention. 2014; 20: 238–243.

101
Mangione TW, Chow W, Nguyen J. Trends in lifejacket wearing among recreational boaters: a dozen years (1998–2010) of US observational data. Journal of Public Health Policy. 2012;33(1):59–74.

102
Szpilman D, Smicelato CE. Quick response to maritime and riverine emergencies in Brazil – a diagnosis of maritime services. World Conference on Drowning Prevention – ILS, Malaysia 2015, Book of Abstract, RESCUE Section, p261. doi: 10.13140/RG.2.1.1933.2568.

103
Smicelato CE, Szpilman D. Rescue crafts operators – reinforcing the use of personal protective equipment. World Conference on Drowning Prevention – ILS, Malaysia 2015, Book of Abstract, RESCUE Section, p267. doi: 10.13140/RG.2.1.1081.2889.

104
Quistberg DA, Bennett E, Quan L, Ebel BE. Low lifejacket use among adult recreational boaters: a qualitative study of risk perception and behavior factors. Accident Analysis and Prevention. 2014;62:276–84.

105
Staines C. History of drowning deaths in a developing community – the Victorian experience. Melbourne: Monash University; 2013.

106
Szpilman D, Avramidis S. Video survey on people's perceptions about the most impactful messages that raise awareness and change attitudes about drowning. In: Abstracts. World Conference on Drowning Prevention, Potsdam, Germany, 2013:78. doi: 10.13140/2.1.2877.1525.

107
Szpilman D. To properly target drowning prevention resources, you need local data: evaluating drowning death data at a local level to understand and plan more appropriately. In: Abstracts. World Conference on Drowning Prevention, Danang, Viet Nam, 2011:119.

108
Frisby ML, Hill JH. A community's response to childhood drownings. A model for accident prevention. Critical care nursing clinics of North America. 1991;3(2):373–379.

109
Rahman A, Miah AH, Mashreky SR, Shafinaz S, Linnan M, Rahman F. Initial community response to a childhood drowning prevention programme in a rural setting in Bangladesh. Injury prevention. 2010;16(1):21–25.

110
Adapted from Schopper D, Lormand JD, Waxweiler R, editors. Developing policies to prevent injuries and violence: guidelines for policy-makers and planners. Geneva: World Health Organization; 2006:5.

111
Gerdmongkolgan S, Ekchaloemkiet S. Policy advocacy on child drowning prevention in Thailand. Conference paper. World Conference on Drowning Prevention, Danang, Viet Nam, 2011.

112
Injuries. In: WHO Health topics [website]. Geneva: World Health Organization; 2016 (http://www.wpro.who.int/topics/injuries/en/, accessed 6 November 2016).

113
Drowning Prevention Report Sri Lanka: Laying the foundation for future drowning prevention strategies. Colombo: Life Saving Association of Sri Lanka; 2014.

114
Thompson NJ, McClintock HO. Demonstrating your program's worth: a primer on evaluation for programs to prevent unintentional injury. Atlanta: Centers for Disease Control and Prevention, National Center for Injury Prevention and Control; 1998.

115
Queiroga AC, Leitão Nuno, Szpilman D. Drowning Science will benefit from research conducted by experienced lifeguards assisted by academics – practical example. In: Abstracts. World Conference on Drowning Prevention – ILS, Malaysia, DATA Section, 2015:25. doi: 10.13140/RG.2.1.4882.3769.

116
Bartolomeos K, Kipsaina C, Grills N, Ozanne-Smith J, Peden M, editors. Fatal injury surveillance in mortuaries and hospitals: a manual for practitioners. Geneva: World Health Organization; 2012.

117
Injury Surveillance Guidelines. Geneva: World Health Organization; 2001.

118
Guidelines for conducting community surveys on injuries and violence. Geneva: World Health Organization; 2004.

119
Verbal Autopsy Standards. In: WHO/Health information and statistics [website]. Geneva: World Health Organization (http://www.who.int/healthinfo/statistics/verbal_autopsy_standards1.pdf, accessed 11 November 2016).

120
Barss P, Subait OM, Al Ali MH, Grivna M. Drowning in a high-income developing country in the Middle East: newspapers as an essential resource for injury surveillance. Journal of Science and Medicine in Sport. 2009;12(1):164–170.

121
Lunetta P, Tiirikainen K, Smith GS, Penttilä A, Sajantila A. How well does a national newspaper reporting system profile drowning? International Journal of Injury control and Safety Promotion. 2006;13(1)35–41.

122
Ghaffar A, Hyder AA, Bishai D. Newspaper reports as a source for injury data in developing countries. Health policy and planning. 2001;16(3)322–325.

123
Szpilman D, Tipton M, Sempsrott J, Webber J, Bierens J, Dawes P et al. Drowning timeline: a new systematic model of the drowning process. American Journal of Emergency Medicine. 2016;34(11)2224–2226.

124
Wallis BA, Watt K, Franklin RC, Taylor M, Nixon JW, Kimble RM (). Interventions associated with drowning prevention in children and adolescents: systematic literature review. Injury Prevention. 2014;21(3):195–204. doi:10.1136/injuryprev-2014-041216.

125
Peden AE, Franklin RC, Leggat PA. Fatal river drowning: the identification of research gaps through a systematic literature review. Injury Prevention. 2016;22:202–209. doi:10.1136/injuryprev-2015-041750.

126
Peters DH, Tran NT, Adam T. Implementation research in health: a practical guide. Geneva: Alliance for Health Policy and Systems Research, World Health Organization; 2013

127
Rubin T. SwimSafe: a survival swimming curriculum. Presentation at the World Conference on Drowning Prevention, Da Nang Viet Nam, 2011.